Xenotransplantation

Science, Ethics, and Public Policy

Committee on Xenograft Transplantation:
Ethical Issues and Public Policy

Division of Health Sciences Policy
Division of Health Care Services

INSTITUTE OF MEDICINE

NATIONAL ACADEMY PRESS
Washington, D.C. 1996

NATIONAL ACADEMY PRESS • 2101 Constitution Avenue, N.W. • Washington, DC 20418

NOTICE: The project that is the subject of this report was approved by the Governing Board of the National Research Council, whose members are drawn from the councils of the National Academy of Sciences, the National Academy of Engineering, and the Institute of Medicine. The members of the committee responsible for the report were chosen for their special competences and with regard for appropriate balance.

This report has been reviewed by a group other than the authors according to procedures approved by a Report Review Committee consisting of members of the National Academy of Sciences, the National Academy of Engineering, and the Institute of Medicine.

The Institute of Medicine was chartered in 1970 by the National Academy of Sciences to enlist distinguished members of the appropriate professions in the examination of policy matters pertaining to the health of the public. In this, the Institute acts under both the Academy's 1863 congressional charter responsibility to be an adviser to the federal government and its own initiative in identifying issues of medical care, research, and education. Dr. Kenneth I. Shine is president of the Institute of Medicine.

Support for this project was provided by The Greenwall Foundation, the Food and Drug Administration (Award No. FDA D66112 00 95 TD 00), the Health Resources and Services Administration (Award No. 103HR941095P000-000), and the Centers for Disease Control and Prevention (Award No. 0009564092). Funds were provided by the National Institutes of Health through the National Cancer Institute (Award No. 263-MQ-436187), the National Institute of Diabetes, Digestive, and Kidney Diseases (Award No. 263-MK-521072) the National Heart, Lung and Blood Institute (Award No. 263-FJ-520288), and the National Institute of Allergy and Infectious Diseases (Award No. N01-OD-4-2139). Additional funds were provided by the U.S. Department of Defense (Award No. N00014-95-1-0920), the Charles River Laboratories, the W.R. Grace and Company-Connecticut, and the Howard Hughes Medical Institute. Additional support for dissemination of this report was provided by The Greenwall Foundation. The views presented in this report are those of the Committee on Xenograft Transplantation and are not necessarily those of the funding organizations.

International Standard Book Number: 0-309-05549-0

First Printing: July 1996
Second Printing: May 1997

Additional copies of this report are available for sale from the National Academy Press, 2101 Constitution Avenue, N.W., Box 285, Washington, DC 20055. Call (800) 624-6242 or (202) 334-3313 (in the Washington Metropolitan Area).

Printed in the United States of America

The serpent has been a symbol of long life, healing, and knowledge among almost all cultures and religions since the beginning of recorded history. The image adopted as a logotype by the Institute of Medicine is based on a relief carving from ancient Greece,

COMMITTEE ON XENOGRAFT TRANSPLANTATION: ETHICAL ISSUES AND PUBLIC POLICY

NORMAN G. LEVINSKY (Chair),* Wade Professor and Chairman, Department of Medicine, Boston University Medical Center

NANCY L. ASCHER, Chief, Liver and Kidney Transplant Services, University of California, San Francisco

ROBERT A. BURT,* Alexander M. Bickel Professor of Law, Yale University Law School

CLIVE O. CALLENDER, Professor and Chairman, Department of Surgery, and Director, Transplant Center, Howard University Medical College

ROGER EVANS, Head, Section of Health Services Evaluation, Department of Health Sciences Research, Mayo Clinic, Rochester, Minnesota

DENISE FAUSTMAN, Director, Immunobiology Laboratories, Massachusetts General Hospital, and Harvard Medical School

RENEE C. FOX,* Annenberg Professor of Social Sciences, Department of Sociology, University of Pennsylvania

JOAN K. LUNNEY, Research Leader, The Immunology and Disease Resistance Laboratory, Agriculture Research Service, U.S. Department of Agriculture, Beltsville, Maryland

MARIAN G. MICHAELS, Assistant Professor of Pediatrics and Surgery, Children's Hospital of Pittsburgh, and University of Pittsburgh School of Medicine

STEPHEN MORSE, Assistant Professor of Virology, The Rockefeller University

KEITH REEMTSMA, Professor of Surgery, Columbia-Presbyterian Medical Center, New York

DAVID ROTHMAN, Professor of Social Medicine and Director, Center for the Study of Society and Medicine, Columbia College of Physicians and Surgeons, Columbia University

HAROLD Y. VANDERPOOL, Professor of History and Philosophy of Medicine, Institute for the Medical Humanities, University of Texas Medical Branch, Galveston

---

*Member, Institute of Medicine.

Staff

VALERIE P. SETLOW, Director, Division of Health Sciences Policy

CONSTANCE PECHURA, Co-Study Director, Director, Division of Neuroscience and Behavioral Health

RALPH DELL, Co-Study Director, Professor of Pediatrics, College of Physicians and Surgeons, Columbia University

YVETTE BENJAMIN, Research Associate

KATHLEEN LOHR, Director, Division of Health Care Services (through February 1996)

CLYDE BEHNEY, Director, Division of Health Care Services (as of February 1996)

LINDA A. DEPUGH, Administrative Assistant

MARY J. BALL, Project Assistant

NANCY DIENER, Financial Associate

Contents

EXECUTIVE SUMMARY 1

1 SETTING THE STAGE 6
  Introduction, 6
  Study Process and Report Organization, 8
  Approaching Questions of Opportunities and Risks, 9
    The Potential Benefits of Xenotransplantation, 10
    Risk: Precedent and Uncertainty, 15

2 ASSESSING THE SCIENCE BASE 17
  Introduction, 17
  Stages of the Immune Response, 18
    Progress in Molecular and Cellular Biology, 21
  Novel Therapeutic Approaches, 26
    Limitations of Immunosuppression in Xenotransplantation, 26
    Modification of the Source Animal, 27
    Modification of the Host, 33
    Modification of the Graft: Encapsulation, 37

3 INFECTIOUS DISEASE RISK TO PUBLIC HEALTH
  POSED BY XENOGRAFTING 39
  Animal Infections and Xenotransplantation, 40
  Basis for Public Health Concern, 42
  Methods of Risk Evaluation, 45
  Detection Methods, 52

Need for a Registry, 54
Summary, 56

4   ETHICS AND PUBLIC POLICY 57
Patients, Ethics, and Society, 57
   Patients' Perspectives, 57
   Informed Consent, 62
   Justice and Fairness Issues: Organ Allocation and Research, 64
   Social Acceptance of Xenotransplants, 68
   Social Acceptance of Infectious Disease Risk, 70
Value and Use of Animals, 72
   Ethical Theory, 72
   History of Social Responses to Xenotransplantation, 75
   A Moderate Ethical Perspective of Xenotransplantation, 77
   Application to Xenotransplantation, 77
Economic Issues Regarding Xenotransplants, 78
   Aggregate Expenditures for Organ Transplantation, 78
   Transplant Procedure Expenses, 79
   Ethics and Public Policy, 80
   Expenditures for Xenotransplantation, 80
   Insurance Coverage, 81
   Impact of Managed Care, 83
   Justice, Fairness, and the Ability to Pay, 84
Reviewing and Monitoring Xenotransplantation, 85
   FDA Regulation of Xenotransplantation, 88
   Current Regulatory Framework, 88

5   CONCLUSIONS AND RECOMMENDATIONS 92

REFERENCES 97

APPENDIXES
A   Workshop Agenda, 103
B   List of Participants, 111
C   Immunosuppression in Allotransplantation, 123

Xenotransplantation

Science, Ethics, and Public Policy

Executive Summary

Xenotransplantation involves the transplantation of cells, tissues, and whole organs from one species to another. Interest in animal-to-human xenotransplants has been spurred by the continuing shortage of donated human organs and by advances in knowledge concerning the biology of organ and tissue rejection. In addition, the development of novel strategies to protect animal cells and tissues from rejection has resulted in experimental application of xenotransplantation to treat a wide range of diseases, including diabetes and Parkinson's disease. The scientific advances and promise, however, raise complex questions that must be addressed by researchers, physicians and surgeons, health care providers, policymakers, patients and their families, public health officials, the news media, and the public. These questions include how to manage the risk to the patient and society at large of animal-to-human infectious disease transmission, how to address special issues related to informed consent and organ allocation, and how and whether to provide adequate resources for research and clinical application of the new technology, among others.

As a result of early discussions within the Institute of Medicine (IOM) Council on Health Care Technology, and with sponsorship from a number of federal agencies and two foundations, the IOM convened a committee in October 1994 to plan a workshop to consider the scientific and medical feasibility of xenotransplantation and to explore the ethical and public policy issues applicable to the possibility of renewed clinical trials of xenotransplantation. Another area of focus was added in response to increasing concern about the potential risk of animal-to-human disease transmission through xenotransplantation. The three-day workshop was held in late June 1995 and involved

1

43 speakers and presenters and more than 200 participants. The workshop focused on three major topics: the science base; the public health risks of infectious disease transmission; and the ethical and public policy issues, including the views of patients and their families. Based on this workshop and additional deliberations, the committee came to specific conclusions and made recommendations, which are outlined here and summarized in detail in the full report.

RECOMMENDATION 1

There is ample evidence for the transmission of infectious agents from animals to humans. Transmitted organisms benign in one species can be fatal when introduced into other species. Because xenotransplants involve the direct insertion of potentially infected cells, tissues, or organs into humans, there is every reason to believe that the potential for transmission of infectious agents (some of which may not even now be recognized) from animals to human transplant recipients is real. Once an infection is established in the recipient, the potential for transmission to caregivers, family, and the population at large also must be considered a real threat. *The committee concludes that, although the degree of risk cannot be quantified, it is unequivocally greater than zero. Hence, the committee recommends that guidelines for human trials of xenotransplantation address four major areas: (1) procedures to screen source animals for the presence of infectious organisms and consideration of the development of specific pathogen-free animals for use in xenotransplants; (2) continued surveillance throughout their lifetimes of patients and periodic surveillance of their contacts (families, health care workers, and others) for evidence of infectious diseases; (3) establishment of tissue banks containing tissue and blood samples from source animals and patients; and (4) establishment of national and local registries of patients receiving xenotransplants. Special efforts should be made to coordinate with international registries and databases.*

RECOMMENDATION 2

The committee discussed various alternatives for oversight or regulation of clinical trials in light of the risk of transmission of infectious agents to the general population from xenotransplantation. Several committee members felt strongly that special regulation of xenotransplant research is not justified because other types of research, including allotransplantation, also involve substantial risks. Other members of the committee argued that the potential for transmission of new infections to humans is a unique risk justifying special regulations. All members of the committee agreed that some mechanism is needed to ensure attention to the risk of infectious disease transmission. The committee was aware of and commends the effort of the Food and Drug Administration (FDA) and the Centers for Disease Control and Prevention (CDC) in developing the first set of guidelines, which are soon to be released but were not final before this report was complete. *Therefore, the committee recommends that adherence to specific national guidelines be required of all experimenters and institutions that undertake xenotransplantation trials in humans. Local institutional review boards (IRBs) and animal care committees, in consultation with outside experts, are appropriate vehicles for review of proposed protocols, provided that they are required to conform to the national guidelines for minimizing and for continued surveillance of infectious risks.*

The committee is well aware that placing authority for the approval of xenotransplantation trials within local IRBs and institutional animal care and use committees (IACUCs) will require an increase in, or augmentation of, the existing capacity of some of these groups. Further, the mandatory adherence to the soon to be released FDA and CDC guidelines would provide the needed safeguards at the local IRB level, which could be overseen through coordinated efforts of the involved Federal agencies (see Recommendation 4) without establishing a complex and, possibly costly, new regulatory structure.

RECOMMENDATION 3

Transplantation of animal organs also raises new ethical and social questions. To assist local IRBs, IACUCs, and society at large to address such questions, *the committee recommends further investigation into the special ethical issues that are raised by xenotransplantation, particularly those related to informed consent in light of the requirement for lifetime surveillance of patients and those related to fairness and justice in allocating organs, as well as research into the psychological and social impact of receiving animal organs on recipients, their families, and members of the society as a whole.*

RECOMMENDATION 4

The committee is aware of and commends the efforts of the Food and Drug Administration and the Centers for Disease Control and Prevention in developing the first set of guidelines for xenotransplantation, which were not final before this report was complete but developed from discussions with other federal agencies and representatives from stakeholder groups. Addressing the multiple areas that require attention, however, will necessitate ongoing review and the cooperation of federal agencies, universities, and the private sector. *Therefore, the committee recommends that a mechanism be established within the Department of Health and Human Services to ensure needed coordination of the federal agencies and other entities involved in development, oversight, and evaluation of established guidelines.*

One mechanism to achieve greater coordination could be the establishment of an advisory committee comprised of representatives of federal agencies and other relevant groups, such as basic and clinical researchers, ethicists, lawyers, and private industry. It also would be important to include patient groups and the public. An advisory committee could be charged to coordinate, *but not to regulate*, research, policy, and surveillance issues related to xenotransplantation and to suggest modifications of the guidelines based on accumulating information from research and clinical trials.

RECOMMENDATION 5

Some scientists who participated in the workshop believe that the risk of infectious disease transmission is high enough to preclude any further human xenotransplantation trials. After considerable discussion of this view and consideration of the issues listed above that will be required to assess the risk of infection, the committee concluded that the potential benefits of xenotransplants are great enough to justify this risk. Hence, *the committee recommends that, when the science base for specific types of xenotransplants is judged sufficient and the appropriate safeguards are in place, well-chosen human xenotransplantation trials using animal cells, tissues, and organs would be justified and should proceed.*

A NECESSARY CAVEAT

Clinical trials with cellular xenotransplants are already under way, and a real danger exists that the commercial applications of xenotransplant technology will outstrip both the research base and the national capacity to address special issues raised by xenotransplantation, including the risk of disease transmission. The committee considered the total expense associated with research and technology development, especially in light of current fiscal constraints. Substantial, stable resources are needed to support research; to perform diverse, well-designed clinical trials; and to maintain patient registries, tissue and serum sample collections, and surveillance for disease in patient populations. *The committee concludes that the potential of xenotransplantation is great enough to justify funding, by federal agencies, private industry, and other sources, of research and other programs (e.g., tissue banks and patient registries) necessary to minimize the risk of disease transmission.*

1

Setting the Stage

INTRODUCTION

Successful human-to-human organ transplants (allografts) are considered among the great medical breakthroughs of this century. The full promise of this success, however, has been limited by chronic shortages of donated, transplantable organs and by difficulties in preventing organ rejection. Although sporadic attempts by modern medical practitioners to transplant or graft animal organs into humans date back to the beginning of this century, xenotransplantation has been systematically studied by the medical community only since the 1960s. These first modern clinical trials of xenotransplants were performed in patients with end stage renal disease. Organ transplantation was—and still is for the most part—the only option for these patients, and the need for donated organs far outstripped the supply. In addition, techniques to provide chronic kidney dialysis were just being developed at the time and were not widely available. Thus, interest in animals as a source of organs re-emerged.

In late 1963 and early 1964, a team at Tulane University led by Keith Reemtsma transplanted kidneys from chimpanzees into six patients, one of whom lived for nine months. By 1974, including experimental surgeries performed by Thomas Starzl at the University of Pittsburgh, about 20 patients had received xenotransplants. Many of these grafts appeared to function normally at first, but soon the grafts succumbed to immune rejection. Patients later died either from graft rejection, with loss of vital function, or from infections resulting from the use of large doses of immunosuppressive drugs. A voluntary moratorium was established by the transplant community in the United States due to poor survival rates and the advent of renal dialysis.

Xenotransplant trials, however, continued in the late 1980s and early 1990s in Sweden, China, and Hungary.

The introduction of new immunosuppressive drugs (cyclosporine and tacrolimus, in particular), improved understanding of graft rejection, and continuing organ shortages were major factors in more recent xenotransplant trials in the United States. In 1985, at Loma Linda University, Leonard Bailey implanted a baboon heart into Baby Fae, a newborn infant who survived four weeks. This case drew attention to several issues: the plight of neonates, for whom organ shortage is even more dire than for adults; the controversy over the ethics of experimenting on a child; the problem of informed consent for a child; and whether the surgeons might have been able to find a human donor.

In the early 1990s, at the University of Pittsburgh, Thomas Starzl transplanted baboon livers into two patients with advanced hepatitis B infection, using special immunosuppressive therapy. A third patient with AIDS was implanted with baboon bone marrow that did not engraft. One of the two liver transplant patients[1] survived 70 days and the other survived 26 days. Both patients died of infection due to excessive immunosuppression. Even though graft failure was not the cause of death, the grafts did not function normally for reasons that are still not understood (Starzl, 1995).

At present, there are no ongoing U.S. clinical trials of solid organ xenotransplants, although an unknown number of proposals are under review. Several clinical trials are proposed or under way with *tissue* xenotransplants for treatment of AIDS or Parkinson's disease, respectively. Cell and tissue xenotransplants, such as pancreatic islet cells or certain types of nerve cells, can encounter a lesser immune response than organ xenotransplants. The reasons for the diminished immune response vary, but include protection of the cells by encapsulation, use of fetal cells that lack immune system "recognition" markers, and separation of the cells from the organ vasculature, the lining of which elicits a strong immune response.

Since the early 1990s, the transplant communities of the United States and many European nations, including Sweden, have not engaged in active clinical trials of xenotransplantation. However, several countries, including Russia, China, and some Eastern European nations, have forged ahead. According to anecdotal reports, hundreds of xenotransplants have been performed in these countries for the treatment of diabetes, using pancreatic tissue from pigs, cows, and rabbits. The magnitude and possible efficacy of these efforts are not

---

[1]One of the patients received a combined bone marrow and liver transplant from the same animal donor. The purpose of the bone marrow was to help engraft the liver by promoting chimerism (the coexistence of human and animal cell populations within the host), a topic described in greater detail in Chapter 2.

known because of poor patient documentation, follow-up, and publication (Ricordi, 1995).

STUDY PROCESS AND REPORT ORGANIZATION

In the early 1990s, informal discussions among the members and staff of the Institute of Medicine (IOM) Council on Health Care Technology suggested that, given the rapidly growing interest in the technology, examination of the science base and ethical implications of xenotransplantation would be appropriate. This report is the result of those early discussions and initial major support from the Greenwall Foundation. Additional support was obtained from the Howard Hughes Medical Institute; the National Institute of Diabetes, Digestive, and Kidney Diseases (NIDDK); the National Heart, Lung, and Blood Institute (NHLBI); the National Cancer Institute; the National Institute of Allergy and Infectious Diseases; the Food and Drug Administration (FDA); the Centers for Disease Control and Prevention; the Health Resources and Services Administration; and the U.S. Navy.

In October 1994, the IOM convened a committee to plan a workshop to examine the scientific and medical feasibility of xenotransplantation and to explore the ethical and public policy issues applicable to the possibility of renewed clinical trials of xenotransplantation. Just before the committee met, another area of focus was added in response to increasing concern about the potential risk of animal-to-human disease transmission (zoonoses) through xenotransplantation (xenoses or xenozoonoses). The committee expanded the workshop to address this issue with additional support from the FDA, NIDDK, and NHLBI. The workshop was held in late June 1995 (see Appendix A) and involved 43 speakers and presenters and more than 200 participants.

This report is based on the deliberations of an expert committee convened by the Institute of Medicine. The committee included clinicians, transplant surgeons, immunologists, specialists in infectious diseases, and social scientists with expertise in health services research, ethics, sociology, and law. The principal source of background information considered by the committee was the workshop it organized. At this workshop 43 speakers reviewed the key areas relevant to xenotransplantation, including the current status of the science base, the infectious disease risk to the public posed by xenotransplantation, and a number of ethical and public policy issues. The presentations were discussed by the more than 200 participants who attended the workshop. The staff also provided the committee with a large number of key articles on the scientific and policy issues relevant to its deliberations. Based on these sources of information and on the expertise of its members, the committee held two day-long meetings at which it discussed and debated the implications of the information for public policy. From these deliberations came the conclusions and recommendations in this report. The body of the report largely incorporates material presented at the workshop, edited for clarity and continuity, and modified and supplemented by the expertise and judgments of the committee. Although the audience for this report is likely to be broad, the committee hopes it will be particularly useful to members of institutional review boards and institutional animal care and use committees that are considering proposals for human trials of xenotransplantation and to policymakers who are charged to participate in the coordination of efforts of the multiple federal agencies involved in xenotransplantation.

The report is organized into five chapters. This first chapter sets the stage by outlining some of the controversial issues that pertain to animal-to-human organ and cell transplants. The next two chapters describe the science base for xenotransplantation and examine the scientific arguments regarding the potential of infectious agents being transmitted to the human population from xenotransplantation. The fourth chapter summarizes the presentations and discussions related to the ethics and public policy implications of xenotransplantation, including consideration of the views and concerns of individual patients and their families. Although Chapters 2, 3, and 4 are based largely on workshop presentations, necessary expansion of background information and key points from committee discussions are included as resources for the reader. The final, brief chapter provides the committee's recommendations regarding the scientific feasibility, ethics, oversight, and regulation of xenotransplantation.

APPROACHING QUESTIONS OF OPPORTUNITIES AND RISKS

All medical innovations, particularly those with the public visibility of xenotransplantation, involve a number of interested groups that are stakeholders in the eventual applications of the innovative developments that ensue. The stakeholders include patients and their families; physicians; scientists; private corporations; public agencies and policymakers; advocacy groups, including patients' rights and animal rights groups; the news media; academics from disciplines such as ethics, law, and economics; and finally, the public at large. Each group is comprised of individuals who hold a variety of viewpoints and beliefs and, thus, are likely to disagree among themselves. In some cases, there are natural partnerships among individual stakeholder groups. In other cases, natural conflicts exist. Some of these partnerships and conflicts are based on key differences in power, investment, organization, and motivation among stakeholder groups. For example, physicians and patients are often partners in medical care and treatment, but when experimental treatment is considered, the patients become research subjects and physicians must take on additional responsibilities as scientists. Doctors who are clinical investigators may face important conflicts of interest between their responsibility as physicians, primarily to the needs of the patient, and as scientists, to the success of the experiment. Although patients are a subset of the public, the two groups can come into conflict when the benefit to one, in this case the patient receiving a xenotransplant, has the potential to harm the other, the public that may be affected by an infection transmitted from this patient or may benefit from a cure.

Public policy must take into account the complex interplay of these stakeholder groups and recognize that this interplay has effects on the development and utilization of new technologies. Xenotransplantation also involves certain key conflicts related to social, moral, and ethical principles. The most prominent conflict involves the willingness of many groups (e.g., physicians, patients, and families) to continue human application of xenotransplant technology, based on the need for better medical approaches to a number of serious human diseases. In opposition, others (e.g., some scientists and government officials) argue that there are significant threats of disease transmission from source animals, threats not only to recipients but to health care professionals, families, and the public at large. A number of controversies about xenotransplantation pose the same kind of need-versus-risk questions, including the use of limited health care dollars. This report will not resolve these questions completely. The committee hopes, however, that the report is useful in identifying some important questions and providing reasonable approaches for the future, within the context of the larger debate and emerging federal guidelines.

The Potential Benefits of Xenotransplantation

Providing Adequate Organ Supply

The case for demand exceeding organ supply could hardly be more stark. According to the United Network for Organ Sharing (UNOS), in 1993 about 33,000 patients who needed organs were on the waiting list;[2] whereas only

---

[2]Once a patient is placed on a waiting list, organ allocation proceeds according to criteria adopted by the board of UNOS after extensive public participation. Allocation criteria include time on waiting list, quality of match for histocompatibility, age of the patient, and medical urgency. These criteria favor the sickest people, including those who require a second or third transplant.

about 7,600 people donated organs (UNOS, 1994).[3] Demand, as defined by the number on the waiting list, grew by more than 100 percent over the five-year period 1988–1993 (Table 1-1). The real need is even higher because many potential recipients, who are too frail or are unable to pay, are not placed on the waiting list (a topic discussed in Chapter 4).

In 1993, approximately 3,000 people died waiting for organs. This number represents a 95 percent increase over the number of waiting list deaths reported in 1988. Not surprisingly, the waiting time for some types of organs almost doubled over the same period. From 1988 to 1992, the wait for kidneys, for example, rose from a median of 360 days to 621 days. The plight of those on the waiting list is best captured by the often-quoted statistic that about 50 percent of those on the list die owing to the lack of a suitable organ.

Although other technologies have been developed to assist patients waiting for organs, none of these achieves optimal results and, often, none is sufficient to prevent death if an organ does not become available. For example, kidney transplant candidates have two options—kidney dialysis and the possibility of receiving a kidney from a living donor. In addition, some patients with heart disease can be aided by left ventricular assist devices. Even these technologies, however, do not obviate the possible benefits of xenotransplantation. Dialysis is only a stopgap measure; it involves dramatic and sometimes long-standing disruption of normal daily life and can, by itself, cause debilitating side effects. The use of left ventricular assist devices confers benefits for an even shorter period than dialysis and negatively affects the patient's quality of life. Both dialysis and assist devices often fail, and patients die before an organ becomes available.

The use of organs, such as kidneys and single lungs, from living donors has increased. For example, a recent study found excellent three-year survival rates (80–85 percent) among patients with kidney disease who received a transplant from a spouse or an unrelated donor, despite a histocompatibility mismatch (Terasaki et al., 1995). Such donations, however, carry varying degrees of risk, pain, disfigurement, and disability for donors. They also raise new social and ethical issues. It is important to note that there are some groups of transplant candidates for whom such donors would not be suitable—infants, for example, for whom the correct size of the transplanted organ is an important factor. In addition, only fetal cells are useful for treating spinal cord injuries or Parkinson's disease, but legal prohibitions in many states prevent the use of human fetal cells.

---

[3]Of this total, the majority were cadaveric donors (4,845) and the remainder were living donors. The total number of organs recovered from these donors reached almost 18,000 because more than one organ can be obtained from each donor.

TABLE 1-1 Size of Organ Procurement and Transplantation Network Waiting List, by Organ at End of Each Year

Organ	1988	1989	1990	1991	1992	1993	1994
Kidney	13,943	16,294	17,883	19,352	22,376	24,973	27,498
Liver	616	827	1,237	1,676	2,323	2,997	4,059
Pancreas	163	320	473	600	126	183	222
Kidney-Pancreas	0	0	0	0	778	923	1,067
Heart	1,030	1,320	1,788	2,267	2,690	2,834	2,933
Heart-lung	205	240	225	154	180	202	205
Lung	69	94	308	670	942	1,240	1,625
Total	16,026	19,095	21,914	24,719	29,415	33,352	37,609

SOURCE: United Network for Organ Sharing Scientific Registry data, 1995.

The National Organ Transplant Act (NOTA) of 1984 established a national network of registries and organ procurement organizations. After the passage of NOTA, the solution to the organ shortage was first thought to reside with increased public education. It seems, however, that public education does not increase the donation rate significantly, because donation has remained fairly stable over time, despite educational efforts and a requirement in more than 25 states for physicians to request organ donation from families of suitable donors. Only about 40 percent of potentially eligible donors are successfully recruited (Siminoff et al., 1995).

The organ shortage has led to numerous other proposals designed to increase donation. For example, some European countries have instituted a policy of "presumed consent" in which organ donation is presumed to be the wish of the patient in the absence of documentation or family statement to the contrary. Yet, this policy does not seem to have resulted in greatly reduced organ shortages. Cash payment for organs is strictly prohibited under NOTA, because many believe that such an approach makes the human body a commodity and, thus, greatly increases the risk of abuse. Other proposals, based on the concept of "rewarded giving," have included, for example, help with funeral expenses. None of these proposals, however, has been accepted or put into operation in the United States. Much publicity has focused on reports from other countries, such as China, in which organs "on demand" have been obtained and sold to the highest bidders by deliberately scheduling executions of prisoners to coincide with a planned transplant. Further, these executions were carried out by using methods that maximized organ viability for transplant. Even if such obvious violations of human rights were isolated or prevented in most countries, there are many in the transplant community who believe that measures to compel or remunerate donation would nevertheless undermine a fragile system that rests on "gifts of life" or voluntary donation for altruistic reasons.

Providing Cells and Tissues to Treat Disease

The second major potential benefit from xenotransplantation is the ability to use cells and tissues from animals to restore the functions of critical physiological systems affected by a variety of diseases. Experiments in laboratory animals and experiments currently under way (mostly outside the United States) with human subjects suggest real promise for xenotransplantation of cells and tissues. For example, clinical trials outside the United States have shown that transplantation of insulin-producing pancreatic islet cells from pigs into humans with diabetes results in nearly normal, and stable, levels of insulin. This would confer an improvement over insulin injections, which result in varying blood levels of insulin over time, because stable levels of insulin in diabetics are important in preventing the devastating side effects of severe diabetes, effects that include blindness, painful neuropathies, hypertension, and life-threatening infections. It is also important to note that the use of pancreatic tissue from humans to treat diabetes is not a suitable option. To provide enough tissue to transplant one person, pancreases from two persons are required and the organ must be "fresh" or taken before death, as in whole organ transplants. Thus, the organ shortage for human pancreases would be even more severe than that for hearts, lungs, and kidneys.

The promise of xenotransplantation of cells and tissues is heightened by the observation that cells and tissues are not rejected as readily as whole organs because strategies have been developed to "protect" the transplanted cells and tissues from the recipient's immune system (discussed more fully in Chapter 2). One of the innovative approaches is to enclose animal cells and tissues in tubes or spheres having holes, or pores, that are large enough to allow passage of physiologically relevant substances—such as insulin—from the cells into the recipient, but are too small to allow passage of immune system cells or antibodies.

Compared with whole organ transplantation, the success of cell and tissue xenotransplantation would potentially provide viable treatments for diseases that affect many more lives. In addition to their use for diabetes, xenotransplants of dopamine-producing neural cells could replace the dopamine cells destroyed in patients with Parkinson's disease. The possibility also exists for replacement of myoblasts in patients with muscular dystrophy. For diabetes and Parkinson's disease, successful methods for cell and tissue xenotransplantation could become a useful therapy if used early in disease progression. Early intervention might yield savings in the required medical care of these patients and decrease losses due to disability.

One proposed human experiment in the United States generated much publicity and debate at the workshop and throughout the preparation of this report. The proposal was to inject baboon bone marrow cells (known to be resistant to the human immunodeficiency virus that causes AIDS) into a person with AIDS in San Francisco. After a long period of review by numerous groups, the patient received the experimental transplant in December 1995 and was still alive in February 1996. By that time, although there was no evidence that the baboon cells had engrafted, the patient's health had improved, as measured by increased numbers of the patient's own white cells, possibly due to an unexpected effect of the radiation used before the transplant to partially destroy his bone marrow.

In summary, the opportunity potentially exists to improve or save the lives of hundreds of thousands of people by development of xenotransplantation. With the success of xenotransplants of cells and tissues already on the horizon, whole organ xenotransplantation has become the subject of renewed investigation. Such potential benefits provide a strong motivation for physicians and scientists to move ahead and for patients to hope. The opportunity to realize these benefits, however, is not without risks, which by themselves provide equally strong motivation to be wary.

Risk: Precedent and Uncertainty

As noted above, the most prominent controversy about whether or not to continue with xenotransplantation involves the possibility that harmful or deadly infectious agents from animals may be transmitted to humans through xenotransplants and could even pose a significant public health threat. Unquestionably, there is ample justification for raising this argument, but there is also great uncertainty over the actual level of risk and how to balance the risks against the potential benefits of proceeding (see Chapters 3 and 4). What is less immediately apparent is how this controversy has changed some of the classic issues that accompany the initiation of clinical trials of any new medical procedure or treatment.

Risk is typically viewed on a highly individual level in clinical trials, and the regulations governing human subjects research reflect this individual focus. These regulations require that a person who agrees to become a research subject be fully informed about the risks of the procedure or treatment before the person consents to participate. The principle of informed consent applied to research subjects has been a key area of study since the Nuremberg trials in the late 1940s, and especially since the emergence of academic disciplines focused on bioethics more than 25 years ago.

The controversy about infectious disease from xenotransplants poses a novel issue in research ethics that will require extensive exploration and public debate. Who can give "informed consent" to a procedure that may cause harm not only to the research subject, but also to many others not directly involved in the research and not direct beneficiaries of success? Will it ever be possible to know the level of risk and to balance it against benefits? Are there ways to manage the risk and prevent harm to others?

Such questions were discussed extensively in the workshop and by the committee. One tentative answer generated before this report was completed derives from approval of the much-publicized trial to use baboon bone marrow cells to treat AIDS. This approval, with numerous special requirements for disease surveillance, was given by the Food and Drug Administration after approval from the Institutional Review Board and the Laboratory Animal Care and Use Committee at the University of California, San Francisco. Far short of an enduring resolution to the questions above, the approval of this protocol nevertheless represents a decision to proceed cautiously and evaluate along the way (Chapman, 1995).

Although most prominent, infection is not the only risk presented by xenotransplantation. For example, some transplant surgeons and others fear that too much publicity about xenotransplantation will decrease public willingness to donate organs, even though the technology is years away from providing a practical resolution of the needs of people who require whole organ transplants. Still others are concerned that clinical practice may forge ahead despite the absence of an adequate scientific base, which happened, for example, with in vitro fertilization.[4] In addition to the adverse effects of immunosuppression and the vascular damage that can accompany allotransplantation, there are risks that xenotransplantation may have negative effects on the quality of life of recipients, despite providing a medically effective outcome. There is also uncertainty about the eventual expense of xenotransplantation—a complex issue that will be a critical determinant of the extent of eventual use of various types of xenotransplantation and must be considered in light of any eventual savings (e.g., decreased health care expenditures for diabetics with xenotransplants of pancreatic islet cells; also see Chapter 4).

Important ethical and social issues regarding xenotransplantation need extensive further consideration. Indeed, some of these issues have not yet been resolved for human-to-human organ transplantation. How will animal and human organs be allocated? Will socioeconomic status influence allocation, so that the affluent and powerful are more likely to receive human organs, while the poor and disenfranchised receive animal organs? Should animals be killed to provide organs? Are there fundamental psychological factors that will lead to problems for recipients of animal organ transplants? People who have received human organ transplants often report having deep and complex emotions about having another person's organ in their bodies. Will this be magnified in people who receive animal organs? Will the expense of xenotransplants outweigh the benefits?

Questions such as these were raised throughout the workshop and in the deliberations of the committee amidst discussion of significant scientific progress and hope for the potential benefits of xenotransplantation. The issue of public health risks, however, clearly dominated and molded these discussions. As a result, the report that follows presents many scientific and ethical issues interwoven with scientific discoveries and hypotheses, which raise both familiar and novel ethical and legal issues at the frontier of medical innovation.

---

[4]The success rate of in vitro fertilization remains only about 20 percent in the best facilities, in part because the growth of the science base has been seriously hampered by political and ethical debates concerning abortion and research on human embryos.

2

Assessing the Science Base

INTRODUCTION

Xenotransplants, or xenografts, are viewed as one solution to the growing problem of the inadequate supply of human organs and as a source of cells, tissues, and organs that show promise for treating a variety of human diseases. This chapter was drawn largely from the workshop Session I: Assessing the Science Base. Thus, the majority of the chapter summarizes workshop presentations. Where useful for background, some sections have been supplemented with additional information. The chapter, however, is not intended as an in-depth analysis and summary of the field of transplant immunology. The committee is aware that there are views of this field other than those presented here and that there are facets of transplant immunology not discussed.

The immunological response to a xenograft depends, in part, on the phylogenetic distance between the source animal and the host. Transplants between closely related species (e.g., example, humans and nonhuman primates or rats and guinea pigs) are called concordant transplants and are less likely to elicit an immediate reaction. However, transplants between more distantly related species, such as those from swine to humans, are called discordant transplants and elicit an immediate immunological reaction that destroys the endothelial lining of the blood vessel of the graft. Transplants of cells and tissues are not subject to immediate rejection since they lack blood vessels. Thus, discordant transplants of whole organs are rejected immediately, whereas such a reaction does not occur with concordant transplants.

For the most part, rejection of a xenograft is more vigorous than rejection of an allograft. Explanations for this are the stronger nature of the immunological responses against xenografts than against allografts and the existence of immunological reactions by the host that are unique to xenotransplantation. Although immunosuppressive drugs are highly effective in allotransplantation, rejection, especially late after transplantation, still occurs. In contrast, immuno-suppressive agents cannot overcome certain aspects of xenograft rejection. It is largely for this reason that investigators worldwide are seeking novel therapies that can supplement the use of immunosuppression to achieve survival of xenografts. New immunosuppressive drugs will also be needed to suppress certain aspects of xenograft rejection. Xenografts of cells and tissues are the first to reach small-scale human trials because means of preventing or blunting the immune response to those transplants are being developed rapidly.

The promise of success of xenografts is derived from research on newer therapies and strategies in animals. Heart transplants from monkeys to baboons (closely related species) have survived for months—some for more than a year. These encouraging results have prompted researchers to propose human trials in which baboon hearts are envisioned as "bridges" for patients awaiting human organs (i.e., as a means of sustaining life until a human donor becomes available). Success has also been achieved with long-term survival of transplanted organs between various rodent combinations (e.g., hamster and rat), but questions remain about the applicability of results of experiments conducted in rodents to human xenografting.

Although the major problem in xenotransplantation is rejection, biochemi-cal and physiological aspects of xenograft function are also unanswered concerns. For example, transplanted bone marrow can react with the heart to cause complications. As new agents are developed and tested, the adverse side effects of those agents will require close monitoring (see Appendix C)

Strategies to counteract human immune rejection of xenografts vary with the tissue or organ being transplanted, the disease being treated (e.g., diabetes, AIDS, or Parkinson's disease), the nature of the transplant (tissues or organs), and the phylogenetic dissimilarity between the patient and the source animal. Both tissues and organs are being modified by either immunological or genetic engineering approaches. Cells or tissues such as pancreatic islets have been encapsulated to deny access to the recipient's immune system. Whole organ xenografts between phylogenetically distant species are the most difficult because a series of new rejection mechanisms, not previously encountered in allograft rejection, must be addressed.

STAGES OF THE IMMUNE RESPONSE

The immunological response to an organ xenograft can be divided into different phases, although the division is to some extent arbitrary, both because the manifestations of one can continue into, or be present in, another and because they can occur as a continuum. The first phase, **hyperacute rejection,** does not ordinarily occur in allotransplants, although in certain situations there can be hyperacute rejection of an allograft if the recipient has certain types of antibodies against the donor cells (Platt, 1995). Current practices detect the presence of such antibodies, and hyperacute rejection is avoided. Hyperacute rejection is a serious problem because conventional immunosuppressive drugs cannot control it. Hyperacute rejection occurs in discordant but not in concordant transplantation.

Each phase of rejection is characterized by the time of its appearance after transplantation and by the rejection mechanisms that seem to be involved (Table 2-1). Hyperacute rejection begins in minutes and results in rejection of the organ within one to two hours in the great majority of cases. If hyperacute rejection is avoided, then the graft is rejected after a period of some days by a process known as **delayed xenograft rejection** (also referred to as acute vascular rejection), which begins within hours and results in rejection after several days (Table 2-1). Although not yet proven, since delayed xenograft rejection has not been completely overcome in a discordant organ transplant model, it is exceedingly likely that the next phase of rejection would involve the xenograft counterpart of a **T-cell (cell-mediated)** immune response that is responsible for rejection of an allograft. Only if all of these phases are overcome does one expect that a discordant organ xenograft may undergo **chronic rejection**, after a period of weeks or months.

TABLE 2-1 Different Types of Xenotransplant Rejection

Characteristic	Hyperacute	Acute (delayed)	Chronic
Time course	Minutes–hours	Days–weeks	Months–years
Type of immune reaction	Humoral	Mostly cellular	Both
Site of action	Blood vessels	Blood vessels or other cells	Unknown
Limiting factor for:	Whole organ xenografts	Organ and cell xenografts	Unknown

Apart from the pace and time of onset, the phases are also distinguishable on the basis of whether the immune response is humoral, cellular, or both. Humoral immunity refers to host responses to an infectious agent or foreign protein by molecules such as antibodies and complement that are found in body fluids. Cellular immunity refers to reactions mediated by whole cells such as T-lymphocytes. Both of these reactions can secondarily involve cells other than T-cells including neutrophils, macrophages, and natural killer cells, which are found in blood and tissues. Hyperacute and delayed xenograft rejection are due primarily to humoral immunity in which preexisting antibodies of the recipient act together with the recipient's complement to initiate the rejection response, although it is hypothesized that other stimuli can initiate delayed xenograft rejection (Bach et al., 1995). Cell-mediated (T-cell) rejection is initiated by T-cells and can involve other cells. The causes of chronic rejection are poorly understood but likely involve both cellular and humoral immune responses.

Hyperacute rejection is a formidable obstacle to successful whole organ xenografting. It is easily recognized clinically because the graft very rapidly becomes swollen and turns black. Hyperacute rejection results from preformed xenoreactive natural antibodies binding to endothelial cells that line the blood vessels of the graft. Endothelial cells stimulated by xenoreactive antibodies plus complement become activated (Bevilacqua et al., 1984; Pober and Gimbrone, 1982). This activation very rapidly results in a profound disruption of endothelial cell integrity and function. Endothelial cells are normally linked tightly to one another to create a barrier that prevents leakage of cells and proteins from the blood into the extravascular space of the organ. Also, endothelial cells normally express, on their surfaces, molecules that prevent clotting and platelet aggregation. When the endothelium is activated, as in hyperacute rejection and delayed xenograft rejection, its barrier and anticoagulant functions are lost, blood cells and fluid leak out into tissues resulting in hemorrhage and edema, and thrombosis occurs in the graft. The sequence of molecular events that culminates in hyperacute graft rejection is described in the section dealing with mechanisms of hyperacute rejection.

Hyperacute rejection is not a factor in cellular xenografts, such as transplants of pancreatic islet cells, because such grafts are revascularized by the recipient; thus, the endothelial cells are self (i.e., not "foreign").

If hyperacute rejection is prevented by depleting xenoreactive antibodies or blocking complement in the recipient, then the graft survives to experience delayed xenograft rejection. This form of rejection also involves endothelial cell activation, but in this instance it appears to be due primarily to up-regulation of new sets of genes on the activated endothelial cells. It is also possible that some of the features of endothelial cell activation associated with hyperacute rejection, which precipitate the earlier thrombosis and inflammation, actually cause delayed xenograft rejection.

Cell (T-lymphocyte) mediated rejection is postulated to be the next phase of the immune response against a discordant organ xenograft. By analogy with allograft rejection, a T-lymphocyte-mediated response in xenograft rejection is initiated when the recipient's T-lymphocytes recognize foreign antigens on the cells of the graft. The antigens recognized are those associated with the major histocompatibility complex (MHC).

Immunosuppressive drugs are used to suppress the T-cell response. For the most part, suppression of this response is quite successful for allotransplantation, although episodes of acute rejection can occur despite immunosuppression. In the nonimmunosuppressed patient, cell-mediated immunity leads to rejection of an organ allotransplant in 7–10 days. If immunosuppression is unsuccessful, rejection of the organ will occur at this time or a little later. A deterioration or change in graft function typically prompts clinicians to suspect acute rejection. Finding immune cell infiltrates in biopsies of the graft is diagnostic. Immune cells can react either with graft endothelium passenger white blood cells (leukocytes) in the graft or with graft parenchymal cells (cells essential for organ or tissue function).

T-cell-mediated rejection, especially that associated with the action of helper (CD4$^+$) T-lymphocytes, involves recruitment and activation of macrophages, plus cytokine-mediated effects on graft endothelial cells. The result is development of graft thrombosis and ischemia due to loss of the anticoagulant molecule, thrombomodulin, and induction of a procoagulant tissue factor that is present on both infiltrating macrophages and graft endothelial cells (Hancock, 1984; Platt, 1994).

Finally, chronic rejection is marked by a slow but progressive loss of graft function that begins months to years after transplantation. Pathologically, graft tissue architecture deteriorates during chronic rejection. Both cellular and humoral immune responses have been implicated but have not been well characterized. Chronic rejection is difficult to manage with conventional immunosuppressive medication and may progress to the point where another transplant is needed. What is known about chronic rejection comes from the study of allografts, primarily because discordant xenografts have not remained viable long enough to meet with chronic rejection.

Progress in Molecular and Cellular Biology

Much scientific progress has been made in defining the molecular basis of hyperacute and delayed xenograft rejection, the first and second phases of the host immune response to a discordant organ xenograft. This understanding allows design of potential therapeutic strategies for overcoming immune rejection.

Mechanisms of Hyperacute Rejection

Hyperacute rejection occurs when vascularized whole organs are transplanted between species combinations that are phylogenetically distant, such as pigs and humans. Hyperacute rejection begins when preformed xenoreactive natural antibodies (which are present at the time of transplantation) in host blood combine with cell surface molecules on graft endothelial cells. The binding of antibodies to these cell surface molecules induces a conformational change in the antibody that exposes a binding site for complement, another key component of humoral immunity. These events on the surface of the endothelium cause the endothelium to lose two critical properties, its barrier and antithrombotic functions. Disruption of the endothelium leads to edema and hemorrhage as blood migrates from the vessel into host tissue. To seal the gaps in the endothelium, thereby stopping blood loss, platelets aggregate and blood clots. These clots obstruct the flow of blood that feeds the graft. Without blood flow, the graft dies.

Although the initial step in this sequence of events is antibody binding to graft endothelium, the subsequent binding of complement is an important event in the immune response (termed an effector function). Although complement is best recognized for its ability to destroy its target by lysing the cell membrane, the role of complement in hyperacute rejection does not appear to be through lysis of the graft endothelial cell. Rather, as discussed below, the role of complement is to induce endothelial cells to change their shape, and thus lose their barrier function, to release several molecules from their surface, including thrombomodulin, heparan, sulfate, and ecto-ADPase (adenosine disphosphatase). These molecules maintain an antithrombotic environment around the endothelial cells. Later, if hyperacute rejection is avoided, complement acts to regulate a large number of genes that contribute to thrombosis and inflammation.

Complement is activated when it binds to an antibody molecule. Host antibodies that bind to the xenograft, xenoreactive antibodies, are mostly of the IgM isotype, one of the five classes of antibodies (the other four are IgA, IgD, IgE, and IgG). The more distantly related the species combination, the higher is the concentration of these xenoreactive IgM antibodies in host blood (Hammer, 1989). Pathology studies using markers that bind to IgM have identified IgM antibodies along endothelial cell surfaces of xenografts; depletion of serum IgM antibodies before transplantation prevents hyperacute rejection.

Recent studies have identified the specific target (epitope) for xenoreactive antibodies on the surfaces of endothelial cells (Cooper, 1995; Squinto and Fodor, 1995). It is a complex molecule, ending in a simple sugar called α-galactose, which is attached to a cell surface protein to form a glycoprotein.

These glycoproteins (those having the α-gal epitope) are found in most mammals, with the exception of apes, Old World monkeys, and humans. Because most nonhuman primates lack these glycoprotein antigens, they form antibodies against the α-gal and thus have the antibodies present before the transplant. The removal of the galactose portion of surface glycoproteins on endothelial cells of pigs reduces the binding of xenoreactive antibodies of primate hosts by 80–90 percent and, thus, also reduces the binding of complement.

These findings are important because binding of xenoreactive antibody to surface glycoproteins activates the complement system and initiates a cascade of enzymatic reactions that can be likened to a domino effect. To understand this cascade, it is essential to point out that complement actually refers to one of several classes of proteins that circulate in the blood as proenzymes (i.e., enzymes whose active site is masked). When one of the complement proteins is activated through antibody binding, it becomes active as an enzyme and causes a change in another complement protein. This reaction generates yet another complement enzyme, which affects yet another complement protein. The multistep process ultimately forms a complex called the membrane attack complex and other intermediary complement products that take part in the immune reaction. Both membrane attack complexes and intermediary products participate in hyperacute rejection.

One complement product (C5a), together with the preformed antibodies, induces endothelial cells to lose heparan sulfate, a substance that prevents blood clotting. This promotes the formation of platelet clots, leading to ischemia. Another complement protein causes changes in the structural integrity of endothelial cells, which leads to gaps in the endothelial surface and subsequent edema and hemorrhage (Platt et al., 1990).

The critical role of antibody binding with subsequent complement activation in hyperacute rejection is supported by experiments in which either xenoreactive antibody or complement is depleted prior to xenotransplantation. These procedures have been shown to prevent hyperacute rejection in that the graft is no longer rejected within hours. In a number of experiments, antibodies were successfully removed by plasmapheresis, immunoabsorption, and other procedures. In another series of animal studies, complement was reduced to nearly undetectable levels before transplant by administration to the host of purified cobra venom factor, which depletes complement. When the whole organ was then transplanted from guinea pigs to rats or pigs to baboons, graft survival was extended from approximately 90 minutes to several days. However, the graft was destroyed after a few days in what is referred to as delayed xenograft rejection (Bach et al., 1995). Cobra venom factor is not a realistic long-term therapeutic strategy for human recipients because of its toxicity and the requirement for continuous infusion. Nonetheless, these studies indicate that techniques that avoid hyperacute rejection may allow the use of xenografts as temporary or bridge measures for patients awaiting a suitable allograft.

Because complement is such a basic part of the host immune system, cells must be protected when complement molecules are activated on their surface. (Complement is usually activated by antibody, as described above, but can also be activated without the participation of antibody.) To protect cells from activated complement, mammals have evolved a number of mechanisms. The most significant mechanism, from the standpoint of potential therapies for hyperacute rejection, involves a group of cell surface proteins called complement regulatory proteins, or regulators of complement activation (RCA). These proteins are species-specific and serve to inhibit complement activation at various points in the complement cascade. The surge in knowledge about complement regulatory proteins and the genes that encode them has spawned a variety of approaches to counteract hyperacute rejection, some of which are discussed in a later section of this chapter.

Mechanisms of T-Cell-Mediated Rejection

Most of our knowledge about T-cell-mediated reactions comes from studies of allografts. Such studies are the basis of the discussion that follows (Faustman, 1995).

T-cell-mediated rejection of organ transplants occurs within days to weeks of transplantation and has been characterized only in allografts. T-cell-mediated rejection is characterized by gradual loss of graft function brought about by a cellular immune response. Host immune cells react with a variety of graft cells, including vascular endothelial cells and parenchymal cells. Humoral immunity may also play a role, but the presence in graft biopsies of cellular infiltrate suggests that cellular immunity predominates.

It has long been known that the response of host T-cells to histocompatibility antigens on the surfaces of cells in the graft is responsible for acute allograft rejection. The detailed molecular mechanisms of recognition and response, however, were poorly understood before the great progress made over the past years in the fields of immunology and molecular biology. Much of this progress has been to identify antigenic determinants, identify how antigen is presented to the host immune system, and identify how the immune system reacts.

Cell-mediated rejection is initiated by activation of host T-lymphocytes (T-cells). T-cells play a pivotal role in controlling the immune response that destroys graft cells. T-cells participate in the activation of macrophages, natural killer cells, B-lymphocytes, and other immune cells. Some of the most effective immunosuppressive drugs in clinical use today work by disabling critical T-cell function (see Appendix C for discussion of desired characteristics of immunosuppressive drugs; based on Kahan, 1995, and Kahan and Ghobrial, 1994).

The graft antigens that most commonly activate host T-cells are MHC Class I and II proteins. These are cell surface markers that not only distinguish one species from another but also distinguish among members of a given species. The amino acid variation in MHC proteins is greater between species than within species, but within-species variability is enormous and elicits an immune response. Put simply, MHC molecules dictate whether the graft is accepted as self or is rejected as nonself. An allograft recognized as self has MHC Class I and II surface markers identical to the host and has a number of other histocompatibility antigens, referred to as minor histocompatibility antigens, that are identical to the host. A mismatch in MHC antigens between graft and host leads to acute T-cell rejection in both allografts and xenografts. The response by the host to foreign MHC antigens is very strong, even stronger than the host's reactions to other foreign antigens, such as viruses and bacteria. Subsequent *in vitro* studies have shown that the response to foreign MHC molecules is greater than that to other antigens by a factor of up to 100 (Kaufman et al., 1995).

MHC molecules are expressed on all cells in the body, although the class of MHC molecule varies. MHC Class I molecules are found on all mammalian nucleated cells, but Class II molecules are expressed on only a few cell types: endothelial cells and immune cells such as B-cells, dendritic cells, monocytes, and macrophages. Accordingly, a graft possesses MHC Class I molecules on all of its cells, but MHC Class II molecules are present only on endothelial cells in its blood vessels and on its passenger leukocytes, which are immune cells residing in any tissue. It is important to understand the distribution of Class I and Class II molecules on the cells of the graft, because their presence or absence determines which type of T-cell is activated. For example, porcine graft endothelial cells have both Class I and Class II molecules on their surface and thereby activate two types of host T-cells, whereas endothelial cells of some other species do not constitutively express Class II antigens.

Xenograft cells having Class I antigens activate host $CD8^+$ T-cells (cytotoxic T-lymphocytes), while those having Class II antigens activate host $CD4^+$ T-cells (helper T-cells). The designations $CD4^+$ and $CD8^+$ refer to molecular markers on the surface of the T-cell. When a $CD4^+$ T-cell recognizes a foreign Class II molecule, it does not directly destroy the target cell, but rather stimulates other immune cells to do so. First, an activated $CD4^+$ T-cell proliferates; then, its daughter cells release intercellular messengers termed cytokines or lymphokines. Cytokines signal B-cells (B-lymphocytes) to differentiate and to secrete antibodies that react with antigens. Cytokines secreted by $CD4^+$ cells also stimulate $CD8^+$ T-cells, macrophages, and other immune cells to destroy a given tissue (Table 2-1). In short, foreign Class II antigens on the surface of appropriate cells activate host CD4$^+$ T-cells that orchestrate an immune response by a variety of immune cells.

MHC Class I molecules are recognized by CD8$^+$ T-cells. When this type of T-cell is activated, it proliferates into a population of effector cells called cytotoxic T-lymphocytes (CTLs), which have the capability to bind to cells carrying the appropriate antigen. It should be noted that xenografts possess other antigens besides Class I and II molecules that are recognized and destroyed by the host immune system, but they do not appear to play as important a role, at least in the systems thus far studied.

How host T-cells recognize foreign antigens has been the focus of much research that has led to the development of immunosuppressive medications. T-cell recognition has been found to be a more complex process than antibody recognition of antigen. Host T-cells can recognize an antigen through either direct or indirect presentation of the antigen. With direct presentation, the antigens on the surface of the graft cells (e.g., Class I and II molecules) are recognized directly by the T-cell. With indirect presentation, in contrast, the antigen must first be processed by another kind of host immune cell: an antigen-presenting cell. After the antigen-presenting cell internalizes the antigen, it displays a fragment of that antigen on its cell membrane in the exterior groove of its Class I or Class II molecule. Thus, the host MHC molecule essentially acts as a guidance system or recognition structure for the T-cell. What is intuitively difficult to grasp is that the antigen is a fragment of the graft's MHC molecule, but the ability to recognize this foreign antigen depends on the fragment being displayed to the host T-cell by the host's MHC molecule. Both indirect and direct antigen presentation take place with xenografts, depending on the species combination and on whether the graft is a whole organ or a tissue.

NOVEL THERAPEUTIC APPROACHES

Limitations of Immunosuppression in Xenotransplantation

Rejection reactions are an inevitable result of all organ and cell transplants, except those between identical twins. Many new immunosuppressive medications have been developed in the past two decades for the treatment of rejection in allotransplantation (see Appendix C). These medications attenuate or slow the immune reactions responsible for rejection, although all too frequently they do not completely abolish them since acute rejection episodes and chronic rejection still occur. Although not without serious side effects, the new generation of immunosuppressive drugs has significantly prolonged graft survival of kidneys, livers, hearts, and combined heart–lung transplants, among others.

Medications successful at treating allograft rejection are being investigated in xenograft research, with mixed results. Some are effective for organ transplants between concordant species, particularly in hamster-to-rat transplants. For discordant organ transplants, there are some data showing that immunosuppressive drugs can maintain the organ in the presence of lowered levels of xenoreactive natural antibodies and can prolong graft survival by a few days through mechanisms that have not been elucidated yet. The major obstacle to solid organ discordant xenografts is hyperacute rejection, as discussed above, which cannot be overcome with immunosuppression.

Clinical experience with xenografts is so limited that it is difficult to forecast the effectiveness of existing immunosuppressives in combating immune rejection. Patients receiving xenografts three decades ago did not have the benefit of today's immunosuppressives. In two patients receiving baboon liver transplants, Starzl and colleagues (1993) administered tacrolimus, corticosteroids, and prostaglandin, a regimen routinely used for liver allografts. To prevent humoral rejection, they added cyclophosphamide, which has broad-ranging effects on many cells. The regimen appeared effective in preventing graft rejection, but left the patients vulnerable to infection, from which they died. It should be pointed out, however, that one of the patients was infected with the human immunodeficiency virus, which attacks the immune system. A compromised immune function prior to transplant does not allow conclusions to be drawn about the efficacy of immunosuppression to prevent graft rejection.

Advances in molecular biology and immunology have suggested new therapeutic strategies beyond immunosuppression to overcome xenograft rejection. The range of approaches can be grouped into three major categories: modification of the source animal, development of chimeras by bone marrow transplantation, and encapsulation of the cells or tissues to be transplanted. The three approaches, their advantages and disadvantages, and their applications to xenografts are discussed below and summarized in Table 2-2.

Modification of the Source Animal

Through modification of animal tissue, investigators can create designer tissues to render them less immunogenic or susceptible to rejection. Tissue is designed or modified by one of several methods that use immunological or genetic engineering techniques. The first method is through masking of antigen with antibodies. The second is through genetic manipulation with transgenic technology, which includes the use of blocking strategies at the RNA (ribonucleic acid) level to stop translation of the antigen or another factor. The

TABLE 2-2 Novel Antirejection Strategies in Xenotransplants

Modification of Source Tissue

Antibody Masking
- Masks surface antigens, such as MHC Class I
- Useful in islet or other cellular xenotransplants
- Blocks acute rejection
- Feasible, but very difficult for application to whole organ transplantation
- Human clinical trials under way using this strategy for Parkinson's disease

Transgenic Modification
- Alters genes for molecules involved in immune responses
- Has been done in pigs to "insert" human gene for complement inhibitors
- Needs a promoter sequence to increase transgene expression in transplant tissue
- Effective, but not sufficient to prevent hyperacute rejection
- Alternative use to insert human transferase enzyme to block formation of epitope on glycoproteins of endothelial cells

Gene Knockout
- Deletes genes coding for antigens that elicit rejection
- Focuses on MHC antigens
- Successful only in tissue xenografts in animal experiments
- Technology severely limited, can be done only in mice

Antisense RNA
- Uses complementary fragment of RNA to bind to native RNA and block synthesis of antigenic proteins
- Technology far from application

Modification of the Host

Bone Marrow Chimerism
- Host bone marrow destroyed and "replaced" by bone marrow of donor or source
- Replaced bone marrow produces immune cells that do not recognize transplant as foreign
- Applied in human clinical allotransplant trials
- Can result in graft-versus-host disease caused by action of T-lymphocytes
- Recent work promising with facilitating cells and removal of T-cells
- Possible use of mixed (donor and host) bone marrow chimerism to decrease risks

Microchimerism
- Recently discovered in long-term transplant survivors and after pregnancy
- Caused by gradual release of lymphocytes and other immune cells from transplanted tissue into host (or mother); enhancement may prolong graft survival

Strategy without Modification

Encapsulation
- Pores in capsules allow cell transplants to release desired biochemicals
- Pores small enough to "protect" cells against immune cells and antibodies
- Pores large enough to allow passage of toxins and viruses from transplant
- Application for diabetes now in human clinical trials
- Pores large enough to allow access of some host cytokines

---

third is through gene knockout technology, which selectively inactivates the gene coding for the antigen or another factor that is involved in rejection. Each of these approaches is described below. The idea of modifying the source animal is to avoid immunosuppression or any other treatment of the host that might be toxic.

Antibody Masking

Antibody masking strives to conceal antigens derived from the source animal from the host's immune system by covering them with antibody fragments. Antigens on the surface of the cell derived from the animal become hidden from cytotoxic T-lymphocytes of the host. This approach has demonstrated success in animals and represents an example of successful xenotransplantation of tissues without the need for immunosuppression. The cardinal studies introducing the concept of designer tissues by donor antigen masking were performed in rodents transplanted with human cadaveric islet cells and liver cells (Faustman and Coe, 1991). Before transplantation, the human cells were treated in vitro with antibody fragments, which shielded the MHC Class I antigens responsible for acute rejection by host cytotoxic T-lymphocytes. Class I antigens were selected for antibody masking because of their expression on islet cells and because of the sparse expression of other epitopes such as ICAM-1 and LFA-3, which on other cell types promote adhesion between host cells and the graft. It was not necessary to mask epitopes responsible for hyperacute rejection, because the islet and liver cells were nonvascularized and, as such, eventually carried endothelial cells of the host.

In these experiments, human islets implanted into rodents survived more than 200 days, without the need for host immunosuppression. Their proper functioning was demonstrated by physiological and histological assays. Liver cells and neuronal cells similarly treated have been shown to survive in xenogeneic experiments in animals. The importance of masking Class I antigens was substantiated by experiments that eliminated (by depleting passenger leukocytes) or masked other immune determinants, such as CD29, which did not result in similar survival in this model system.

Success with antibody masking of Class I antigens in xenotransplantation experiments in animals has led to human clinical trials. Antibody-treated fetal pig neurons rich in dopamine are being transplanted into the brains of patients with Parkinson's disease.

Source animal modification through antigen masking has proved effective with cells and homogeneous tissue such as islets in a few selected models tested to date. Source animal modification is also feasible, although far more difficult, for whole organs (Faustman, 1995). Not only do whole organs contain a multiplicity of cell types with a variety of antigenic determinants, but organs also contain vascular endothelial cells foreign to the recipient and, thus, are complicated by hyperacute immune rejection. Therefore, alternative strategies have been developed for modification of organs, including the production of transgenic animals (i.e., animals that express an additional gene introduced by genetic methodology).

Transgenic Modification

The production of transgenic organs also has potential as a strategy to shield animal organs (and tissues) from rejection by humans without the need for immunosuppression and represents another form of source animal modification (Squinto and Fodor, 1995). The source organ can be modified at the genetic level before implantation. Genes that are important to prevent rejection can be added through transgenic technology. In transgenic modification, either all cells of the animal contain the foreign gene (transgene) which is incorporated stably into their genome expressing the protein, or only selected cells contain it due to the use of promoters (genetic elements that control expression of a gene) that are specific for a single cell type. The transgenes most commonly used to date in xenograft research molecules that inhibit the human complement cascade, and are thus, intended to block hyperacute rejection.

The idea of creating transgenic donors that express human inhibitors of complement was proposed by Dalmasso and Bach (Bach et al., 1991; Dalmasso et al., 1991). These investigators showed that incorporating human decay-accelerating factor (DAF) (which blocks the complement cascade), at the stage of C3, into porcine endothelial cells in vitro blocked the ability of the human complement to lyse the porcine endothelial cells. They based their suggestion for creating such transgenic pigs on the fact that complement inhibitors such as DAF are species-specific; therefore, the porcine DAF present in the endothelial cells of a porcine organ that is transplanted to a human would not effectively inhibit human complement and would not prevent hyperacute rejection. Thus, the human gene DAF should be expressed in source animals by microinjection of the gene into the nucleus of a fertilized porcine egg by conventional transgenic technology.

Such manipulation gives rise to a mature source animal that incorporates the transgene into the genome of all cells. The mere presence of the human gene for DAF in every cell of the source animal does not, however, ensure its expression at levels high enough to inhibit complement. High level are required, particularly on the surface of source animal endothelial cells, where complement is activated. Therefore, a promoter DNA sequence that boosts the level of expression of the transgene is attached to the human DAF gene. The hope in these experiments is that high enough levels of expression of human DAF will be achieved in porcine endothelial cells to block complement action. It appears that transgenic source organs that express human DAF are not rejected hyperacutely, at least in some cases.

Another gene encoding an inhibitor of complement that has been used to make transgenic source animals is CD59, which inhibits the final reaction in the complement cascade (i.e., formation of the membrane attack complex). Studies of the efficacy of transgenic organs expressing human CD59 have yielded mixed results. Porcine hearts, kidneys, and lungs that express human CD59 have been transplanted into Old World monkeys. These recipients are similar to humans insofar as they carry preformed antibodies causing hyperacute rejection of porcine organs. After transplantation, transgenic organs survived up to 48 hours, a significant improvement over nontransgenic organs, which survived only about an hour. The use of transgenic animals expressing inhibitors of complement may succeed in inactivating complement proteins, but it does not prevent binding of preformed antibodies. Although it was originally thought that the binding of preformed antibodies was benign as long as the ensuing complement attack was arrested, further research suggests that the binding of preformed antibodies does more than just activate complement. Antibody binding to the vascular endothelium of the xenotransplant, by itself, can cause deleterious changes in the endothelial cell (Platt, 1994). An alternative approach to blocking hyperacute rejection is by abolishing expression of the galα(1–3)gal epitope that is recognized by preformed antibodies in the host on the graft endothelial cells, an idea proposed by Sandrin McKenzie and colleagues (McKenzie et al., 1995), and others. This idea is being tested by inserting a gene that causes fucose instead of galactose to be added at the end of the carbohydrate chains, yielding the carbohydrate surface marker found on universal donor, or O blood group, cells. This fucose-containing surface glycoprotein does bind the xenoreactive antibodies. One research team has developed a transgenic mouse cell line that over expresses the enzyme, human transferase (H-transferase). This enzyme competes with the one that catalyzes placement of the galactose at the end of the carbohydrate chain, thereby reducing the formation of the α-galactose antigenic epitope on the surface glycoprotein and blocking hyperacute rejection. Herds of transgenic pigs and mice expressing H-transferase are currently being produced to determine the utility of this approach for transplantation to humans.

Gene Knockout

Another technique from molecular biology that can be used to modify a donor organ is referred to as gene knockout technology (Koller, 1995). It is used to inactivate a given gene(s). In theory, gene knockout can be used to delete permanently from animal organs and tissues genes for any antigens or other factors that elicit rejection. To date, gene knockout technology has been limited to use in mice.

Thus far, investigators have concentrated on inactivating the complex of genes associated with the expression of MHC Class I antigens involved in rejection. Knockout animals have been used to study both tissue and organ allografts, but only tissue xenografts. Knockout mice have also been created that do not make β2-microglobulin, a protein that forms an integral part of Class I antigens. Kidneys and liver cells from these knockout mice have prolonged survival when implanted into other mice; liver cells implanted into frogs also fared well, without immunosuppression.

Development of technology that could allow gene knockouts in pigs or other species suitable for organ donation to humans would represent a major step forward in xenotransplantation. Embryonic stem cell lines, needed for all current approaches to create knockouts (see below), have not yet been established for these higher species. When gene knockouts are developed for these other species, it would permit, for example, inactivation of the gene encoding the enzyme that is responsible for forming the antigenic epitope on surface glycoproteins, thereby potentially blocking hyperacute rejection. T-lymphocyte-mediated rejection could perhaps be avoided by disabling the set of genes encoding Class I or II MHC antigens. In short, advances in knockout technology could lead to the creation of xenogeneic organs that could bypass rejection by human recipients.

An even newer version of gene knockout technology is capable of inactivating the gene in selected cell types, such as T-lymphocytes or endothelial cells. In standard knockouts, the gene is inactived in all cells, which can be lethal. With the new technology, gene inactivation can be restricted to certain types of cells, allowing, for example, selective elimination of MHC Class I and/or Class II antigens on specific cells, such as endothelial cells.

Antisense RNA

Antisense RNA is a therapeutic strategy aimed at preventing expression of a given gene in the graft. It is designed to block the translation of functional gene products into protein antigens by the incorporation of antisense oligonucleotides—synthesized messenger RNA (mRNA) sequences that are complementary to, and thus hybridize with, specific mRNA sequences responsible for protein synthesis. Once hybridized to the proper native mRNA, antisense RNA interrupts the synthesis of selected proteins in the graft. However, antisense RNA is a technique that appears to be more complicated than originally thought and is far from realization for xenotransplantation.

Modification of the Host

Bone Marrow Chimerism

Bone marrow chimerism represents another strategy to circumvent the immune response in either allotransplantation or xenotransplantation (Ildstad, 1995). The strategy calls for bone marrow to be transplanted into a host along with a solid organ from the same donor or source animal, or from a second donor carrying the same antigens as the first. Bone marrow engraftment may confer permanent acceptance of organs and tissues from the same source or donor without the need for immunosuppression, a state called tolerance. The host is described as a chimera because its bone marrow contains cells from both source or donor and recipient. Bone marrow chimerism has been shown to induce tolerance in studies of allotransplants and xenotransplants in rodents, and clinical trials with allotransplants in humans are under way.

Bone marrow is the source of many types of immune cells and, hence, is a major part of the immune system. In bone marrow transplantation, source or donor bone marrow can essentially replace the host's immune system with that of the source or donor, and the immune cells produced by this reconstituted bone marrow do not reject tissue or organs from the donor, since those tissues or organs are seen as self. For this strategy to work, the host's immune system must first be destroyed with radiation and/or chemotherapy, an extremely high-risk procedure. In contrast to modification of the source animal, bone marrow transplantation represents modification of the host. The host undergoes more than just immunosuppression: the host's immune system is either entirely or partially destroyed and replaced with transplanted cells. The justification for giving radiation and/or immunosuppression is to make room for the graft, although recent research suggests this may not be needed. At least for allotransplants, if the donor marrow engrafts permanently, long-term immunosuppressive medication is very likely no longer necessary.

Bone marrow chimerism has been studied in both humans and animals for decades, but recent progress has laid the foundation for human clinical trials of bone marrow implantation in patients requiring allogeneic or xenogeneic whole organ transplants (described later). Experiments in animals in the 1950s revealed that allotransplants of skin would not be rejected if they were accompanied by bone marrow or spleen transplants from the same source animal. However, a skin transplant from a genetically different source animal was rejected. The problem was that recipient animals later died, mostly likely from graft-versus-host disease (GvHD).

GvHD, a serious complication of bone marrow transplantation, is caused by immune cells from the graft recognizing the host as foreign or nonself. It can occur either in bone marrow transplants alone or in combination with organ transplants using either allogeneic or xenogeneic tissue. Graft leukocytes initiate an immune response that rejects host tissues, most commonly skin, gastrointestinal tract, and liver. The host immune system does not reject the immune cells of the graft because host cells have been destroyed by pretreatment with radiation and/or cytotoxic drugs. Even today, GvHD is lethal in 15 percent of the patients who develop it after allotransplants of bone marrow, and approximately 50–70 percent of all bone marrow transplant patients show some symptoms of GvHD.

A major research goal of the past decade has been to understand GvHD. After determining that GvHD was caused by mature donor T-cells, investigators used donor marrow depleted of mature T-cells in several human clinical trials. However, the remaining bone marrow cells did not engraft in up to 70 percent of these patients, a lethal complication for those patients whose own bone marrow had been totally destroyed. Because of these results, GvHD was thought to be an unavoidable complication of bone marrow allotransplants, rendering the prospect for bone marrow xenotransplants even more remote.

Recent research in rodents, however, has yielded evidence of a new cell type in bone marrow that acts to facilitate engraftment in allotransplants and xenotransplants of bone marrow. The insight came from experiments showing that syngeneic bone marrow grafts (grafts from the same or a genetically identical individual) were successful, even if T-cells were depleted. Yet the same graft of purified bone marrow cells did not engraft in genetically different individuals of the same species (allografts). Suzanne Ildstad reported at the workshop that she and her colleagues (Kaufman et al., 1994) reasoned that the purification process had inadvertently removed a population of cells that helped or facilitated engraftment across histocompatibility barriers. They referred to these as facilitating cells. Facilitating cells comprise less than a half a percent of total bone marrow cells and must be matched genetically to the bone marrow donor. As few as 30,000 of these cells ensure engraftment of allogeneic and xenogeneic marrow that is devoid of mature T-cells. With facilitating cells, donor marrow reconstitutes an immune system in the host without causing GvHD. Facilitating cells administered without other marrow cells do not engraft. These cells share some surface markers with T-cells, which explains why they were removed when the marrow was purged of T-cells. However, they do not perform some of the conventional functions of T-cells, at least in part because they do not have T-cell receptors on their surface. How facilitating cells aid in engraftment is not yet known.

Facilitating cells have been shown to be effective in promoting bone marrow chimerism in a variety of animal species with allografts and xenografts. Researchers also have discovered that complete ablation of the host's immune system may not be necessary for bone marrow chimerism to succeed. Partial ablation carries the distinct advantage of a lesser risk.

To produce a functioning immune system, transplanted bone marrow cells must mature, and some of the mechanisms of this process have been discovered. It appears that some bone marrow cells from the source or donor, known as stem cells, migrate to the host's thymus, the normal site of development of certain immune cells. In the thymus, the source or donor stem cells destined to become T-cells undergo a process of maturation and selection. It is at this site that they are thought to become tolerant to the host.

Clinical trials are under way at several transplant centers to determine the effectiveness of allogeneic bone marrow transplants along with transplants of kidneys or livers. In at least one trial, bone marrow is depleted of mature T-cells, leaving behind stem cells, progenitor cells, and a putative facilitating cell population. In another trial, two unmodified bone marrow infusions are given separately to increase the dose of marrow (Ricordi, 1995). The degree of destruction of the hosts' immune systems varies between trials. In some, patients receive partial instead of complete ablation of their immune system; in others, no ablation is undertaken. If any of these clinical trials prove successful, allogeneic bone marrow transplants may have applications to immune and autoimmune disorders. Indeed, this evidence led to proposals for human trials with xenogeneic bone marrow, including the controversial clinical trial discussed at the workshop and performed later that year, which involved transplant of baboon bone marrow into an AIDS patient.

Over the last decade David Sachs, Suzanne Ildstad, and their colleagues have tested a mixed chimerism approach in which bone marrow from the donor is given together with host bone marrow (Ildstad, 1995). This procedure allows a lower dose of irradiation to be used and has the advantage of more fully reconstituting immune function in the recipient than does total replacement of the bone marrow with only allogeneic bone marrow. This procedure shows promise for permitting survival of xenografts with less loss of immune competence. The application of bone marrow chimerism to solid organ discordant xenografts would require additional steps to circumvent hyperacute rejection.

In summary, establishment of bone marrow chimerism represents a high-risk, high-reward strategy for whole organ allografts and, potentially, xenografts. The high risks are incurred when the patient's immune system is destroyed, or severely impaired, to make way for the donor marrow. The procedure also carries the risk of GvHD, but this risk may be reduced by depletion of mature T-cells from the donor. Bone marrow offers the tantalizing prospect of permanent acceptance of allogeneic whole organs without the need for long-term immunosuppression, and likely would contribute to the survival of a discordant xenograft.

Microchimerism

Another strategy that could be employed to increase host acceptance of whole organs is microchimerism, which is caused by the migration of leukocytes out of the graft and dispersion throughout the host. The patient becomes chimeric, as defined by the coexistence of foreign and host cells, but only at a microlevel because of the small number of donor cells present in the host.

Microchimerism occurs naturally after transplantation. It also occurs naturally after pregnancy, as was discovered by obstetricians who found fetal cells in maternal serum, sometimes years after pregnancy. The existence of microchimerism after transplantation was discovered only recently by Thomas Starzl and his group at Pittsburgh with the advent of better detection technologies, such as use of the polymerase chain reaction (PCR). Hypotheses about its role in graft acceptance came from studies of long-term survivors of kidney transplants. Patients who survived transplants from the 1960s were examined in the early 1990s. Biopsies revealed donor cells throughout host tissues, although few in number. The presence of donor cells in a host years after transplantation meant that cells of donor origin were not destroyed by the host immune system. The identification of coexisting immune cell populations in healthy transplant recipients led Starzl and his colleagues to propose that microchimerism is a desirable, rather than an undesirable, consequence of transplantation that ought to be fostered. It also is seen as a predictor of graft success. These investigators hypothesized that the two-way communication between graft and host leads to a state of mutual tolerance, which can occur only under what they term the protective umbrella of immunosuppression. If the balance is tilted too far in either direction, GvHD or rejection of the graft will occur (Starzl et al., 1993). Once mutual tolerance occurs, immuno-suppression should in theory no longer be necessary. To promote microchi-merism, these and other investigators are infusing bone marrow cells at the time of whole organ transplant in ongoing clinical trials.

Modification of the Graft: Encapsulation

Encapsulants are semipermeable barriers designed to surround transplanted cells to protect them from the host's immune response. The foreign cells or tissues, either allogeneic or xenogeneic, are placed in a polymer sheath having pores that are selectively permeable to molecules of low molecular weight. The pores are impermeable to immune cells and large molecules, including antibodies and complement if desired. The pores are sufficiently large, however, to permit passage of such molecules as insulin and other hormones, growth factors, and other molecules of small molecular weight. The encapsu-lated cells survive and function because the pores allow uptake of oxygen and nutrients from blood and interstitial fluid, and they allow exit of waste products. Encapsulants are feasible only for cells and tissues, not for organs. Because of the size of organs, interior cells would die from lack of nutrients if transplanted in an encapsulated form.

Encapsulants are versatile enough to shield a variety of secretory cells, but much of the research by industry and academic investigators has focused on encapsulating islet cells, including those from the pig, for the treatment of human diabetes. Insulin secreted by pig islets is nearly as effective as human insulin and has enjoyed widespread clinical use for decades. Islet cells are superior to insulin for regulation of blood glucose levels because injections do not achieve the fine control over glucose levels needed physiologically. This lack of fine control leads to serious and debilitating complications such as atherosclerosis of larger vessels and painful neuropathies. Besides this therapeutic advantage, encapsulated cells offer other advantages: they are only minimally invasive; the biocompatible encapsulant sheath is durable and, if large enough, can be retrieved along with its contents in the event of rejection or dysfunction; and because the encapsulated cells are shielded from cellular rejection, the recipient should require little or no immunosuppression. *Unencapsulated* islet allografts encounter immune cellular rejection and therefore require immunosuppression of the patient.

What remains to be demonstrated is whether encapsulants can protect against the cytokine-mediated autoimmune damage that caused the disease in the first place, since cytokines can enter freely through the membrane.

Cytokines are believed to play a key role in diabetes because they are directly toxic to islet cells. Type I diabetes involves a poorly understood autoimmune process in which the immune system reacts to autoantigens from islet cells, and destroys the cells. Encapsulated cells likely release some (porcine) islet antigens, which are seen as foreign by the host and lead to T-cell activation with release of cytokines that are of small enough molecular weight to diffuse into the encapsulant.

Problems that must be considered even if encapsulants are used include the following. The pores in the encapsulants are large enough to permit the exit of toxins from infectious agents in the donor tissue (either of allogeneic or xenogeneic origin), if such agents are present in the tissue. Without access to the encapsulated tissue, the host's immune system cannot destroy the tissue harboring the infection. Prescreening potential donor tissue for infections would decrease this possibility, but as noted in Chapter 3, previously unexpected infections may still be present. Another possible disadvantage of encapsulation may be eventual immune reaction to the encapsulant itself. Years of research have been devoted to identifying the best mechanical design for encapsulating cells. Early animal studies placed islets in a relatively large plastic chamber surrounding a shunt that was connected to an artery. This approach failed because the islets died when coagulated blood blocked the pores or the host suffered life-threatening clotting complications such as stroke. Newer approaches with smaller devices have employed hollow fibers and microspheres. To prevent cell clumping inside the capsule, which deprives internal cells of nutrients and oxygen and thereby leads to cell death, the cells can be suspended in alginate or other types of matrix that immobilize them. The matrix does not block the passage of small molecules.

Success with glucose regulation in allograft animal models has led to human clinical trials, in which islets from human cadavers were microencapsulated in hollow fiber devices and implanted into nonimmunosuppressed diabetic patients (Scharp et al., 1994). Over the course of the two-week-long safety trial, no complications were recorded and 90 percent of the encapsulated cells survived. Because there was no detectable short-term immune response, immunosuppression was unnecessary. Insufficient numbers of islet cells were transplanted to draw any conclusions about the efficacy of the procedure, but further trials are planned. If allogeneic tissue proves successful, xenogeneic islet cells are the obvious next step since they are easier to harvest and in plentiful supply. Human pancreases, like other human organs, remain in short supply.

3

Infectious Disease Risk to
Public Health Posed by Xenografting

This chapter was drawn largely from the workshop Session II: Infectious Issues. Thus, the majority of the chapter summarizes workshop presentations. Where useful for background, some sections have been supplemented with additional information. The chapter, however, is not intended as an in-depth analysis and summary of the field of animal-to-human infectious diseases. The possibility that infections can be transmitted from animals to humans is of concern not only because of the threat to the health of the recipient, but also because such infections may be transmissible to others, creating a public health hazard. Further, such infections may be due to previously unrecognized organisms, making detection difficult if not impossible. If the time from infection to clinical symptoms is long, the risk of widespread transmission is greater, because during this time the new organism may silently spread from person to person, as happened with human immunodeficiency virus (HIV).

Emergence of a new public health risk appears to be a two-step process (Morse, 1995). First, a new infectious agent is introduced into a given human population from other human populations, animals, or environmental exposures. Frequently these new agents are zoonoses, defined as animal microbes that can infect humans as well as the animal species from which they come. The second step is establishment and dissemination of organisms that prove to be infective and transmissible from person to person. The first step, introduction of a potentially transmissible agent into a human, could be accomplished by transplanting an organ that was infected with the agent. It is the second step of establishment and dissemination, however, that raises public health concerns, particularly if the agent is viral since current therapies for viral illnesses are limited.

Four questions can help to analyze these potential public health concerns (Chapman, 1995; and Chapman et al., 1995). First, is there reason to believe a patient can be become infected by xenotransplantation? If so, the second question is whether such infections constitute a threat to the general public health rather than a complication limited to the individual xenotransplant recipient. Third, what options are available for the prevention and control of infectious diseases associated with the use of xenogeneic tissue in humans? Fourth, which are the most appropriate options for xenotransplantation?

ANIMAL INFECTIONS AND XENOTRANSPLANTATION

Infections are a major cause of morbidity and mortality after all transplant procedures (Michaels, 1995). They were the cause of serious complications after xenotransplantation in the 1960s when chimpanzee and baboon kidneys were transplanted in two series of experiments carried out by Keith Reemtsma and Thomas Starzl. Bacterial diseases were major contributors to the deaths of five of six of the patients in each of these series. The bacterial infections most likely arose from the recipient's natural flora, but whether infectious agents from the source animal were involved was not investigated.

Consideration of the infectious risks associated with allotransplantation provides some information relevant to xenotransplantation. The major risk factor for infections in patients who receive allotransplants is immunosuppression, which hampers the patient's ability to mount a normal immune response to an infection. Latent infections in the recipient may also be reactivated during immunosuppression. On the other hand, previous infection with an agent no longer present in the recipient can be a resistance factor because the patient may have protective antibodies. The specific organ being transplanted influences the type of infection anticipated. For example, patients who receive a liver have a high incidence of abdominal infections; patients who receive a kidney are susceptible to genitourinary tract infections; and patients who receive a lung or a heart transplant are predisposed to infections of the pulmonary system.

The source of the infectious agents is likewise important. The source of infection can be endogenous flora of the recipient such as skin contaminants that can traverse the skin barrier because of incisions or central catheter lines. Likewise, the source can be endogenous latent infections that might reactivate, such as those caused by *Mycobacterium tuberculosis*, or members of the herpes viruses family. Nosocomial infections can also be transmitted by health care workers or family members that come in contact with the patient. Opportunistic infections with organisms that are in the environment such as aspergillus or legionella are other potential types of infection. Neither the patient's endogenous flora nor the microbial environment will be affected by the source of the transplant (human or animal). However, some infections after allotransplantation are recognized as being from the donor organ or accompanying hematopoietic cells and are especially pertinent to xenotransplantation. Donor-associated infections are usually due to latent microbial agents, although occasionally infections occur due to unrecognized, recently acquired, and active bacterial or viral infections in the donor or source animal. Latent organisms do not cause symptoms in the donor and thus will not be recognized unless specific tests to detect them are employed. The herpesviruses cytomegarovirus (CMV) and Epstein-Barr virus (EBV) are the most frequent donor-associated infections. Other herpesviruses, such as herpes simplex virus (HSV) or varicella-zoster virus (VZV), are usually latent in nervous tissue and, therefore, are less likely to be transmitted by a transplanted organ. HIV, hepatitis B virus, and hepatitis C virus have been transmitted by organ transplantation but are less common now that donors are screened carefully to identify seropositive individuals and remove them from the donor pool. Creutzfeldt-Jacob disease (a disease causes by prions) also has been transmitted by transplantation of human tissues. Parasites can be transmitted by transplantation. For example, *Toxoplasma gondii* has caused infections, particularly after heart transplantation.

In light of this experience with allotransplantation, it is evident that there are several mechanisms by which a recipient could be infected by an organism present in the source animal. The organism could be one that is pathogenic for both humans and animals such as *T. gondii*. An animal virus could be so similar to the analogous human virus that it is able to bind to human cell receptors and cause disease. An agent that is not infectious in normal humans might cause disease in immunosuppressed organ recipients.

Immunosuppression inhibits the development of specific antibodies, thereby increasing the risk of infectious disease for the patient and also hindering some of the usual methods for detecting infectious disease. Recombination of an animal virus from the transplanted organ with a human virus present in the recipient, although perhaps unlikely to occur, is still of concern because such an event could produce a new virus with more pathogenic properties. The actual risk of human-to-human transmission of agents acquired from animal organs, tissues, or cells is not known but is clearly not zero.

It is important to consider the microbial status of the source animal and how the animal was raised. Was the animal in a specific-pathogen-free environment, a quarantined colony, or a farm? What methods were used to screen for specific pathogens?

The pathogenic potential of any zoonotic infectious agent is a function not only of the organism, but also of an evolutionary adaptation between pathogens and their natural hosts. Therefore, the pathogenic potential of an infectious agent can be modulated unpredictably when the microbe is transmitted from its natural host into another species. For example, cercopithecine herpesvirus, or B virus, has a clinical profile in its natural host, the macaque monkey, that usually does not cause disease—similar to the course of herpes simplex infection in humans. However, B virus infections of humans or other nonmacaque primates (due to a scratch or bite from a macaque) can cause neurologic disease that has a mortality rate of approximately 70 percent. Similarly, pseudorabies virus, the pig herpes simplex-like organism, is benign for adult swine but causes fatal neurologic disease when transmitted to a number of other species. Adult pigs and baboons, the animals most commonly considered as sources of cells, tissues, or organs, are almost universally positive for herpesviruses unless raised under special conditions. Additionally, most adult baboons are positive for another organism, foamy virus. Whether these organisms might have more pathogenic potential when transmitted from their natural host across species lines with xenotransplantation is not yet known.

BASIS FOR PUBLIC HEALTH CONCERN

The second question is whether xenogeneic infections constitute a threat to the general public health or are only a complication of the risk–benefit calculation for the individual xenotransplant recipient (Chapman, 1995; and Chapman et al., 1995). Historic experience with many zoonotic diseases suggests that the potential for human infection with xenogeneic pathogens has implications for the community that extend beyond the individual transplant recipient. Although not all zoonoses can be transmitted from person to person, many noteworthy outbreaks have occurred.

For example, in Germany in 1967, importation of vervet monkeys infected with the Marburg virus resulted in a primarily infected human transmitting the virus to another human, ultimately involving 31 persons and a case fatality rate of 23 percent. In Zaire in 1976, the hospital admission of a single patient infected with Ebola, another zoonotic filovirus, resulted in a large nosocomial outbreak that extended into the surrounding communities. Four successive waves of human-to-human transmission were documented, involving more than 200 persons, with a case fatality rate of 88 percent. Most of this transmission occurred in the hospital and between close family members.

In Pakistan in 1976, a shepherd with gastrointestinal bleeding due to infection with Crimean Congo hemorrhagic fever (CCHF), a zoonotic bunyavirus from domestic animals, underwent an exploratory laparotomy for what was presumed to be peptic ulcer disease. Human-to-human transmission ensued, involving 17 persons and a case fatality rate of 24 percent.

These examples demonstrate that some zoonotic infections have the potential to extend beyond the individual and into the community. Thus, the risk of xenotransplant-associated infection is not restricted to the xenotransplant recipient alone. The potential for xenogeneic infections to be transmitted through human populations is real and poses a public health concern. Further, the risk for health care workers in close contact with the xenograft recipient is probably higher than for the community at large.

The initial drama of a zoonotic outbreak predicts the likelihood that it will receive attention but does not predict its eventual public health importance. In fact, the public health consequences of a xenogeneic infection may be most significant when the immediate pathogenicity is least evident. The filovirus and bunyavirus outbreaks were very dramatic, but their public health impact was limited because the infections had a short incubation period and were easily identified, enabling prompt initiation of public health measures to control them. Other infections with very long incubation periods are less easily controlled. For example, initial infections in humans with HIV-1 during the 1970s or earlier resulted in more than a decade of insidious transmission before AIDS was even suspected as a public health problem for the first time in the 1980s. Arguments exist to suggest that the HIV epidemic in humans resulted from a simian retrovirus introduced across species lines into human hosts, where it adapted and was then transmitted (Allan, 1995b). Several species of African monkeys carry an HIV-like virus called SIV (simian immunodeficiency virus) that is part of the animal's normal microbial flora and apparently nonpathogenic in its normal host. Many genetically distinct SIVs have been isolated and named according to the different monkey species in which they are found. Humans have two distinct HIVs, HIV-1 and HIV-2. It is hypothesized, based on molecular biological evidence, that HIV-1 was derived from SIV found in chimpanzees. One interpretation is that only two cross-species transmissions into humans created an epidemic that now has infected 18 million to 20 million people. In some areas of Africa, up to 30 percent of sexually active persons are infected. Stronger molecular evidence supports the idea that HIV-2 was derived from SIV in sooty mangabey monkeys. In addition, the geographic distribution of the HIV-2 epidemic in West Africa among humans parallels the natural habitat of the sooty mangabey.

SIV has been proven to be transmissible to humans. An active and ongoing SIV infection in a human who was working with nonhuman primates has been confirmed by evidence of seroconversion and persistent seropositivity with increasing antibody titers, identification of the seroreactivity of new viral gene products over time, and isolation of the virus from the infected person (Khabbaz et al., 1994). This human SIV infection is not an isolated event. An anonymous serological survey of primate workers demonstrated antibodies to

SIV in 3 out of 472 tested. Not only is there nonhuman primate to human transmission of SIV, but when captive nonhuman primates are housed together, horizontal transmission of retroviruses across species lines occurs on occasion.

The potential for the introduction of a new retrovirus into human hosts via implanted xenogeneic tissue is of public health concern due to the long period of clinical latency associated with all known human retroviral infections. This long latency period provides the opportunity for silent person-to-person transmission to occur before pathogenicity is evident. The pathogenic potential of exogenous retroviruses such as SIV and the baboon simian T-lymphotropic viruses (STLVs) are of concern because they are genetically similar to human exogenous retroviruses HIV-2 and HTLV (human T-cell lukemia virus). The genetic relatedness of humans to nonhuman primates may make transmission more likely with xenotransplants from primates than from more disparate species such as pigs. Some observers consider the use of baboons as a source of organs to be especially dangerous for this reason (Allan, 1995a,b). However, retroviruses are not limited to primates and have been found in many other animals including horses, minks, and cats, with an unknown potential for causing disease in humans.

All eukaryotic species examined, including baboons and pigs) have been found to harbor endogenous retroviral-like DNA (deoxyribonucleic acid) sequences that pose uncertain risks. Endogenous retroviruses are retroviruses that are fixed in the germ line and transmitted as part of the genetic inheritance of the offspring. In the host species, the retroviruses commonly are clinically benign and defective, but some are known to be xenotropic: the virus does not replicate in the host species but is capable of infecting related species. Endogenous retrovirus proviral DNA can be detected in the tissue of all animals examined thus far, including humans, nonhuman primates, and pigs. Baboon retrovirus can be isolated from baboons by cocultivation with human cells. Although no true recombinant of animal endogenous retrovirus with other animal viruses has been described, phenotypic mixing between different viruses can occur under appropriate experimental conditions, which suggests that this and other endogenous retroviruses may have pathogenic potential under conditions associated with xenotransplantation.

Safety generally has been presumed to be increased when swine tissue is used, rather than tissue from nonhuman primates. Swine retroviruses have, nevertheless, been identified, although they are still incompletely characterized. The potential for retroviruses that are latent in porcine tissue to infect an immunosuppressed human host, to rescue replication-defective viruses, or to recombine with latent viruses to create a hybrid is unknown. Further, swine harbor other infectious agents, some of which are known human pathogens. Therefore, the use of swine for xenotransplantation is not without infectious risk.

There are concerns that xenogeneic viruses may recombine or reassort with viruses latent in human tissues and result in variants that possess either a broader host range or an increased pathogenic potential. For example, the periodic emergence of new pandemic influenza strains is thought to occur by a process of reassortment between animal and human influenza viruses. In addition, the oncogenic potential of animal DNA viruses introduced into immunosuppressed humans remains undefined, although cross-species infections do exist. Indeed, one needs to ask whether a pig producer who has received a pig organ xenotransplant could be a source of a novel virus if his transplant were to become infected with a pig virus at the same time that the rest of his body was infected with a similar human virus. If viral recombination occurred, he might (or theoretically could) inadvertently pass this new variant to his own pigs. Thus, a new infection could arise in pigs, causing an emerging swine health problem, in addition to the potential human health problem. Finally, few data exist on the presence in potential animal organ sources of prion-associated disease, similar to Creutzfeldt-Jacob disease or bovine spongiform encephalopathy (Allan, 1995a,b). Prion disease, not yet described in pigs tissue, is of concern, for example, in applications using pig neuronal tissue in parkinsonian patients.

METHODS OF RISK EVALUATION

It is clear that the potential for infectious hazards exists with xenotransplantation. Controlling the risks to human health posed by various hazards is a four-step process involving research, risk assessment, risk management, and risk communication. First, evidence must be collected on the effects of exposure to a particular microbe by an individual and a population. Second, a risk assessment must be performed that includes three related activities:

1. Hazard identification determines if the microbe actually causes an adverse effect.
2. The relationship between exposure and an adverse effect must be determined (i.e., the threshold dose for infectivity).
3. Exposure assessment determines transmissibility of the infectious agent and the number of people likely to be exposed.

A complete risk assessment provides an estimate of the incidence of an adverse effect in a given population.

The third step is risk management, which is the development of guidelines, rules, and regulations. This step should include evaluation of the effects of various approaches in terms of their impacts on public health and on economic, social, and political factors, including a cost–benefit analysis.

Further, risk management may have to proceed in the absence of a complete and quantitative risk assessment. Finally, there should be risk communication, which involves communicating in clear, ordinary language to the affected population and to political leaders, media, and other spokespeople, the results of the risk assessment detailed above. Such communication involves relating relative risk and likelihood to common experience as exemplified by the statement "It is safer to fly than it is to drive a car the same distance."

Regarding the infectious disease risk to public health posed by xenotransplantation, data are missing on several of the links required to perform an adequate risk assessment. The information summarized in the first portion of this chapter permits identification of some of the known potential hazards and has shown that transmission of microorganisms occurs with xenotransplantation from animals to humans. However, hazard identification is incomplete because there are almost certainly viruses present in the animal that are potential human pathogens and that have not yet been identified. Further, some viruses have been detected, such as those in the spumavirus family (foamy viruses), that constitute an uncertain hazard because to date no disease has been linked to the presence of foamy virus in an individual. Neither the number of organisms (threshold) nor the mix of various organisms required to produce a disease in the patient is known. Exposure assessment involves consideration of the presence or absence of various organisms in the animal that was the source of the cells, tissue, or organs; the route of transmission of the microbe; and the types of contacts between the patient and other people. In many cases, it is difficult—if not impossible—to quantitate all of these factors. Thus, quantitative risk characterization is not possible given the current state of knowledge, and risk management will have to proceed in the absence of complete characterization. Risk communication is also difficult because of the lack of data and certainty. Thus, risk management depends on professional judgment, and the public should be informed that the management plan represents a best guess for minimizing risks. Participation of the public in setting guidelines will be important.

What options are available for risk management of xenotransplant-associated infectious public health risk? One option is to eliminate all risk by avoiding all use of xenogeneic tissue in humans. This option, however, would mean the death of many patients each year who are eligible for transplantation, but for whom there are no human donors available and for whom xenotransplants might be effective. Another option would be to dismiss all concerns with risk in the name of medical progress—an option that is unacceptable in light of the considerable data indicating the existence of a public health risk. A different option, which the committee found preferable, is to seek a balance between concerns for public health risks and concerns for desperately ill patients who may be aided by progress in xenotransplantation. This approach requires performing a risk characterization by estimating, to the extent possible, what risks to the public health may exist and then utilizing the risk management tools available to decrease or contain those risks.

The first available tool is pretransplant screening of animal sources of the cells, tissues, or organs for known zoonotic pathogens. The risk of infecting the recipient with previously recognized zoonotic pathogens can be controlled by adequate survey of the animal source, by screening and quarantine the individual animal or developing well-characterized source colonies where feasible, and by attending to the circumstances and methodology of tissue retrieval. Screening should also be performed on the recipient pretransplant (baseline) and after transplant. Posttransplant prospective surveillance of the patient for the occurrence of symptoms suggesting infection and for the presence of microbes in cultured body fluids should be conducted. Both health care workers and family contacts should be followed to detect the occurrence of disease. Finally, tissue from both the animal and the recipient should be archived for future use.

The animal organ source should be screened for known zoonotic organisms that are infectious for humans, such as *Brucella* and *Erysipelothrix* in swine, or organisms that can be present in swine or baboon, such as *T. gondii*, encephalomyocarditis virus, lymphocytic choriomeningitis virus, and Mycobacterium species. Also, screening should be conducted for types of organisms that could be transmissible or could recombine in humans, such as herpesviruses or retroviruses.

Laboratories should use methods of virus testing that are species specific (e.g., baboon specific for baboons) when available and should consider the use of broad range polymerase chain reaction as discussed in the next section on detection methods. It is undesirable to rely on tests that were devised for human viruses because these methods may be insensitive and may miss important viruses in the animal that is to be the source of transplant material. For example, in screening baboons for viruses that might be of concern after xenotransplantation, reasonable concordance was found between two laboratories using antibody tests for cytomegalovirus as well as for simian agent 8, a baboon herpesvirus, but significant discordance was found when looking for evidence of Epstein-Barr-like virus (*Herpes papio*). These two laboratories relied on detecting baboon *H. papio* by cross-reacting serology with human reagents. One laboratory that had very few positive tests utilized an enzyme-linked immunosorbent assay (ELISA) test directed against human EBV nuclear antigen (EBNA). However, recent studies (Michaels and Simmons, 1994) have shown that baboon *H. papio* EBNA 2 is quite different from human EBNA, which may explain the lack of cross-reactivity. The other laboratory relied on an immunofluorescence antibody test directed against the EBV viral capsid antigen, which is a much more conserved portion of this virus. This experience highlights the need to develop tests that are specific for organisms in the animal rather than relying simply on cross-reactivity. Again, it is important to note that nearly all adult male baboons, if not raised in a quarantined environment, are positive for three herpesviruses (simian agent 8, cytomegalovirus, and *H. papio*) and for foamy virus.

When nonhuman primates such as baboons are to be sources of the transplanted material, they should be screened for other organisms that, although unlikely to be found in animals raised in captivity in the United States, would preclude their use as a source of organs. Examples of such organisms include Ebola, Marburg, and Reston, as well as viruses that cause simian hemorrhagic fever and monkey pox. There should also be screening for the retrovirus family of including lentiviruses such as SIV, oncoviruses such as STLV, and simian retrovirus (SRV), as well as spumaviruses (foamy viruses). Many virologists and infectious disease specialists agree that the presence of lentiviruses or oncoviruses should preclude the use of an animal as a source of organs. There are also some who would exclude primates that carry spumaviruses, although these viruses have not been associated with disease even in infected humans.

It is important to look for organisms that are unknown by performing a broad array of viral cultures on a number of different cell lines. A comprehensive strategy for culturing viruses should be developed. This strategy could include establishing cell lines from the animal organ, induction of latent viruses in such a cell culture with inducing agents, and coculturing with a variety of sensitive indicator cells. Any viruses that are found should be preserved so that they can be used at a later date for surveillance purposes when following the patients prospectively. Bacterial stool cultures should also be performed to identify pathogens that have the potential for systemic infection; for example, *Salmonella* species, *Yersinia* species, and other potential pathogens that might have been in the gastrointestinal tract. Blood cultures of the animal should be obtained well in advance of the transplant. This is difficult to do in human donor transplantation but can be accomplished readily in xenotransplantation because the surgical procedure can be planned in advance. Appropriately stained smears of the animal's blood could also be examined for the presence of parasites and intracytoplasmic inclusion in addition to culturing the blood. At the time the organ is harvested, a full necropsy should be performed and, ideally, a number of tissues should be sampled and cultured. Blood and tissue samples should also be archived for surveillance purposes.

Potential recipients should be screened serologically for prior exposure to infectious agents, and serum samples from the patients should be stored to use as pretransplant infectious controls. Recipient surveillance protocols should involve serial serologic screening and viral cultures. Intensive culturing should be employed for fever evaluations. Finally, all biopsy and autopsy specimens should be archived.

Public health guidelines exist that are intended to minimize the risk of transmission of known pathogens by human-to-human transplantation, and similar guidelines are under development that address xenotransplantation. In addition, when human infections with known zoonotic pathogens occur, standard diagnostic testing procedures and disease descriptions may be helpful. Likewise, therapeutic options are available for many of these pathogens. The intense immunosuppression of patients undergoing xenotransplantation may complicate the task of posttransplant monitoring, and of clinical disease recognition, by decreasing the dependability of diagnostic antibody testing and perhaps by altering disease presentation or response to therapeutic intervention. However, immunosuppression will not alter either the culture techniques or molecular diagnostics needed to identify the pathogen or the control interventions available to reduce person-to-person transmission once the infection is recognized.

One method for decreasing the infectious risk posed by xenotransplantation is to use specific-pathogen-free (SPF) animals as a source of transplant material. However, there are several difficulties with this approach. It is critical that SPF be defined for each animal: that is, what pathogen is the animal certified to be free of and what methods were used for the certification? It is not possible to have completely pathogen-free animals, even those derived by cesarean section, because some potentially infectious agents are passed in the genome and others may be passed transplacentally. Gnotobiotic animals (raised in germ-free conditions) are as free of pathogens as possible, but still would have endogenous viruses and might have other transplacentally transmitted organisms. In addition, gnotobiotic animals are very expensive to maintain and, in the case of swine, do not thrive. Raising primates in gnotobiotic environments has not been attempted. Likewise, it would be very expensive and time-consuming to produce an SPF colony of baboons because these animals have a relatively long generation time (they reach sexual maturity in five to seven years). In addition, cesarean-derived animals must be reared in isolation, which is labor intensive, and such a colony would require new, isolated housing facilities separate from other baboons. Animal welfare issues raised by rearing animals in isolation would require considerable attention, and mature animals would have to be trained in the care of newborns for the successful creation of an SPF colony. However, SPF baboon colonies could be achieved. It has been estimated that it would take 7 to 10 years and cost approximately $8 million to $10 million to produce a baboon colony large enough to provide 100 SPF baboons per year. If this approach is taken, animals should be certified to be retrovirus free (except for endogenous retroviruses) and herpesvirus free.

Production of swine that could be used for transplantation would be easier because they become sexually mature in six months and have a four-month gestation time, producing a litter of 3 to 13 offspring, so that after sexual maturity, two litters per year would be possible (Swindle, 1995). These animals grow rapidly, reaching a size suitable for adult transplantation in three to six months. SPF is a term that is currently defined in swine husbandry to denote freedom from certain specified pathogens. Under the current system, herds of SPF swine are raised on farms and are inspected every 90 days to ensure adherence to standards. Vaccination of swine is not allowed if the herd is to receive the SPF designation. However, such swine are a good place to start to develop animals suitable for transplantation purposes. It would probably not be necessary to derive swine by cesarean to establish a pathogen-free herd, because vaccines exist for many swine diseases and there are no rules prohibiting vaccination while developing such a herd for xenotransplantation. A pathogen-free herd would most likely be housed under conditions approaching laboratory animal housing instead of usual farm conditions, although the location of the facility and personnel access procedures would be important concerns as well as the SPF surveillance program.

Six colonies of SPF rhesus monkeys have been developed (Keeling, 1995). These animals are free of SIV, SRV 1–5, STLV, and cercopithecine herpesvirus 1 (B virus). This definition does not include several viruses known to infect nonhuman primates such as spumavirus, herpesviruses other than B virus, adenovirus, reovirus, and spongiform viruses, or other organisms such as *T. gondii*. These animals are in general too small to be useful in human transplantation and may be too phylogenetically distant from an immunological point of view. Production of these animals, with a relatively limited definition of SPF and shorter times to sexual maturity than baboons, takes five years and is expensive—each 2-year-old SPF animal costs about $3,000 (Keeling, 1995). In 1995, non-SPF baboons cost approximately $1,500.

In summary, SPF baboons would not be entirely free of infectious agents, would be expensive to produce and maintain, would require considerable time to develop, and would be an economically stressed approach to decreasing the infectious disease potential of baboons at present. If further research shows that baboons are a good source of cells, tissues, or organs for xenotransplantation, it may be worth reconsidering the production of pathogen-free baboons. Producing pathogen-free swine (the term xenografic-pathogen-free or XPF has been proposed) is feasible (although they too will not be entirely free of infectious agents) and has been done in several areas of the country. The biggest challenge with swine will be to develop immunological strategies to prevent rejection. Transgenic swine that may produce tissues and organs that are better tolerated by the human are being developed (see Chapter 2).

It is the potential for human infections with xenogeneic pathogens not previously described or not previously recognized to pose hazards to human hosts that is of greatest public health concern. Public health surveillance, the primary prevention tool applicable to all emerging infections including risk from xenotransplantation, is useful here. Such surveillance involves ongoing monitoring of a population (recipients and contacts) for events of public health concern, tracking the trends in the rate of occurrence of those events, investigating the causes of any observed increase in trends, and instituting public health interventions combined with continuous monitoring to document further changes in the rate of occurrence of those events after the intervention.

According to a 1992 Institute of Medicine report,

> The key to recognizing new or emerging infectious diseases, and to tracking the prevalence of more established ones, is surveillance. A well-designed, well-implemented surveillance program can provide the means to detect unusual clusters of disease, document the geographic and demographic spread of an outbreak, and estimate the magnitude of the problem. It can also help to describe the natural history of a disease, identify factors responsible for emergence, facilitate laboratory and epidemiological research and assess the success of specific intervention efforts. (p. 2)

Most public health surveillance systems monitor for discrete and definable adverse health events. However, public health surveillance for infections with new or newly recognized pathogens, which may be associated with xenotransplantation in humans, requires monitoring for the unknown. Two questions arise: (1) How can surveillance be conducted for what is not known or recognized? (2) How can the significance of the outcome of such surveillance be assessed?

Xenotransplant recipients will all have underlying illnesses that set them apart from the normal population prior to transplantation. In this setting, surveillance must monitor for adverse health events that are unexpected, unexplained, possibly infectious, and occurring at a higher than normal rate, which is difficult to determine for a distinctly abnormal population. What surveillance approaches are most appropriate to use in xenotransplantation? Surveillance of populations of xenotransplant recipients for clustering of adverse health outcomes and monitoring of individual recipients for unexplained illnesses are probably the most useful public health tools available. This is particularly true in the case of xenotransplantation, because the patients will be identified and surveillance can be focused on these known individuals and their contacts.

There are no standard diagnostic tests available to detect infections with previously unrecognized pathogens. In addition, antibody monitoring is hampered by the immunologic suppression that is required in transplantation. Standard culture techniques may not identify new xenogeneic pathogens. Identification of such pathogens will require the use of a variety of methods that are new or being developed (see section on detection methods below). As an example of the difficulties associated with culturing techniques, in 1976, when a group of attendees at the American Legion convention died in Philadelphia from Legionnaire's disease, it took more than five months of intensive effort before *Legionella* was cultured for the first time.

Surveillance should also focus on those most likely to become infected by an organism from the patient, such as hospital staff or close personal contacts of the patient. The types of organisms that may be transmitted by transplanted tissue are likely to be transmissible through blood or through secretions. Hence, universal precautions should be strictly enforced in all patient contacts. Archiving serum taken from hospital staff and from other people who come in contact with patients posttransplant should be required.

DETECTION METHODS

The concern for xenozoonoses leads to the need to develop carefully validated methods that are both sensitive enough to detect known infectious agents and specific enough to distinguish whether an organism is of human or animal origin (Persing, 1995). Sensitive tests that may be of low specificity can be used to screen for a range of etiologic agents. Traditional methods include electron microscopy to identify structures similar to known pathogens, search for cytopathology in cell cultures inoculated with material suspected of carrying a microbe, and injection of material into animals. Many nucleic acid-based methods developed over the past decade can be quite sensitive and useful in detecting new infectious agents and monitoring infection with these agents. These methods include shotgun cloning, polymerase chain reaction (PCR), representational difference analysis (RDA), sequence-independent single primer amplification (SISPA), and others that are being developed in this rapidly changing field. Some of the more conventional techniques, such as culture and animal model to create a registry recovery techniques, and the technological framework for some of the nucleic acid techniques are discussed below.

Improvements in culture techniques have resulted in the recovery of many organisms not detectable with standard methods, including *Legionella pneumophila, Bartonella henselae, Borrelia* species, *Mycobacterium genevensii*, and other pathogens. These improvements are important advances because, even though nucleic acid techniques are very useful for identifying and characterizing organisms, only by recovery of an organism in culture can it be characterized both immunologically and biochemically. Microorganisms have been recovered by injecting material from animals into immunodeficient rodents, such as SCID (severe combined immunodeficiency) mice infused with portions of the human immune system (SCID-hu mice). Such techniques have permitted recovery of human organisms not capable of growing in normal rodents, such as *Plasmodium falciparum*, Epstein-Barr virus, and *Schistosoma mansoni*.

A nucleic acid technique called representational difference analysis RDA, based on subtractive hybridization, has been developed.[1] The RDA technique has been used to identify several organisms including human herpesvirus 8, which is associated with Kaposi's sarcoma, and a new hepatitis-associated flavivirus. This technique can be used to sort out nucleic acids in a complex mixture and to identify unique sequences that are associated with pathogenic organism. It is a very powerful technique likely to have broad application in identifying not only bacteria, fungi, and protozoa, but also endogenous retroviruses and other viral or novel pathogens.

Another nucleic acid technique is broad-range PCR, which is based on amplifying sequences that are common to a wide variety of species of microorganisms within a phylogenetic family. This technique has been used to identify a broad range of species within a given family: *Rickettsia* species, *Bartonella* species, *Babesia*, *Mycobacterium genevensii*, *Mycobacterium* X, lentiviruses, various human papilloma viruses, and hepatitis viruses. Broad-range PCR depends on the development of PCR primers that can identify

---

[1]In this technique, nondiseased tissue is used as the driver, and diseased tissue containing both normal genomic DNA and DNA from the pathogen is used as the tester. The principle of the method is that the driver is used to subtract normal human DNA from the tester, leaving only the DNA of the pathogen. The steps of this method are as follows: DNA from both tester (or diseased) tissue and driver (or normal) tissue is cut up by a restriction enzyme. The two samples are modified, and oligonucleotide primers are added to both populations of DNA. These primers are then used for amplification of all the DNA within the two different populations of DNA molecules. Once amplified, the two samples are combined after oligonucleotide primers have been added to the tester, or pathogen-containing, DNA. Then a subtraction step or a hybridization step is carried out, yielding self-annealing nucleic acid molecules from the pathogen and molecules that are hybrids of normal tissue DNA and diseased tissue DNA. The only molecules in this mixture capable of amplifying logarithmically (in PCR or a similar amplification technique) are the nucleic acid fragments from the pathogen because these fragments have primers at both ends while the hybrid mixture of nucleic acid molecules has primers only at one end. A 10-million-fold enrichment of the unique DNA sequence occurs after four rounds.

highly conserved ribosomal sequences common to many or all members of a viral family. Species-specific regions in the ribosomal sequences are then identified by using species-specific primers. This method, if automated, might become a routine test in clinical laboratories and permit the identification of a wide range of microorganisms, including uncultured microorganisms. Broad-range PCR could even lead to a new scheme for characterization of microorganisms in which an uncultured organism is identified and phylogenetic analysis is performed. In this scheme, the closest relative that can be grown readily in culture or in an animal is selected on the basis of phylogenetic testing. Serologic reactivity to this available organism is then determined. Such a procedure could permit epidemiologic and seroprevalence surveys for a new organism in baboons or swine that are to be the source of tissue for xenotransplants. Another by-product of this approach is that useful scientific information on infectious agents and the diversity of their natural relatives is likely to result.

One major drawback of PCR-based methods for diagnostic and discovery purposes is contamination. The sensitivity of the method will permit the detection of exquisitely small amounts of contaminating material present in the original sample along with the desired sequence. This key problem can be overcome through rigorous technique, appropriate use of controls, and corroborative methods.

The ideal virology and microbiology laboratory supporting a program of xenotransplantation should combine standard approaches to diagnosis using specific, validated tests and state-of-the-art research methods, which would be sensitive and designed to detect potential pathogens. Such a laboratory should be capable of screening for a long list of known animal and human microorganisms and would be useful in examining posttransplant patients with fever or other symptoms or signs that suggest infection or in evaluating clusters of adverse outcomes. Some workshop participants felt that a central national laboratory should be established to develop and validate new tests and methods. The other option would be to develop collaborative arrangements between laboratories at various institutions.

NEED FOR A REGISTRY

In order to follow patients and their contacts carefully for potential development of infections that present public health hazards, it will be critical to create a registry (Chapman, 1995). A xenotransplantation national registry would collect data on xenotransplant recipients that permitted documentation of significant commonalities among them. Such a registry ideally should be able to capture patients' records automatically and electronically, while safeguarding patient identity. Key clinical and laboratory data about every xenotransplant recipient in the United States would be updated periodically with responses to a standard set of health screening questions and laboratory assays. Because it is necessary to maintain such a registry to protect the public health, prospective xenotransplant recipients would be required to give informed consent to surveillance, most likely for the rest of their lives. Some types of safeguards must be considered for this mandatory lifelong surveillance, however, because it implies the need for enforcement under some circumstances and presents the possibility of limitations to individual freedom and privacy.

Such a national or international registry would allow prospective monitoring of individual xenotransplant recipients and of the recipient population as a whole, as well as retrospective tracking of epidemiologically linked recipients for investigation of adverse events, if they should occur. As another benefit, the registry would allow research on other aspects of xenotransplantation, such as the effectiveness of various immunosuppressive regimes. Archiving of biological specimens from both animals and patients prior to and following the transplants would allow retrospective laboratory investigation of new agents if unexplained illnesses arise.

Investigations of individual instances of unusual illnesses can be revealing, although usually a cluster of cases must occur before a problem can be recognized, a new etiologic agent identified, or associated risk factors delineated. For example, although scattered individual cases had occurred throughout the country for more than a decade, the AIDS epidemic was not even suspected until the spring of 1981 when similar sexual activity histories were noted among seven young men with *Pneumocystis carinii* pneumonia (PCP) in the Los Angeles area. Other examples of cluster investigations that have resulted in public health breakthroughs include John Snow's historic research on cholera in London in the 1850s, which led to the identification of a contaminated water pump as a source of the urban outbreak. Study of a group of patients with pneumonia at the Bellevue Stratford Hotel in Philadelphia led to the identification of the *Legionella pneumophila* organism in 1976. Investigation of the 1993 cluster of unexplained respiratory deaths in the Four Corners region of the United States identified hantavirus pulmonary syndrome. The cost of each of these public health breakthroughs should not be underestimated. When the Minnesota State health department reviewed the results of more than 500 cluster evaluations, 6 of which involved full-scale investigations, only one had resulted in documentation of an outcome of public health significance.

Identifying the causative infectious agent is only one step toward the control of its transmission. Public health threats have been minimized through identification of, and education regarding, risk associations, for example, the association of Reye's syndrome in children with aspirin consumption. Often public health control measures can only decrease, not eliminate, risk. In the relatively controlled xenotransplant setting where exposure is known to have occurred and where there is prospective monitoring, adequate surveillance may be able to detect new xenogeneic infections in recipients prior to significant spread into the general population. Such early detection would allow suspension of the specific procedure, source animal species, or factors associated with risk, pending the development of adequate methods for prevention and control, thereby reducing the risk of additional infections. However, as noted previously, infectious agents such as HIV, which produce clinical disease only after long latency periods, may spread widely in the population before they are detected.

SUMMARY

To answer the four questions posed at the beginning of this chapter:

1. Is there a basis for concern regarding xenogeneic infection for individual human recipients? Yes.

2. Do these concerns constitute a threat to the general public health, rather than being only a complication in the risk–benefit calculation for individual xenogeneic tissue recipients? Although there is considerable debate about the degree of risk, most infectious disease experts agree that some level of risk to the general public health exists.

3. What options are available for the prevention and control of infectious public health risks associated with xenografting in humans? Preplanned transplantation screening of the animal that is the source of the graft for known zoonotic pathogens and posttransplantation surveillance of the recipient for adverse health events possibly associated with xenogeneic infections are the best tools available.

4. What approaches are most appropriate for xenotransplantation? A national xenotransplant registry would permit continuing surveillance of recipients for the occurrence of unusual illnesses. Archiving of appropriate biologic specimens from both the animal source and the recipient would be the key to retrospective investigation of the occurrence of such events.

4

Ethics and Public Policy

This chapter was drawn largely from the workshop Session III: Ethics and Public Policy. Thus, the majority of the chapter summarizes workshop presentations. Where useful for background, some sections have been supplemented with additional information. The chapter, however, is not intended as an in-depth analysis and summary of the complex issues of ethics and public policy related to xenotransplantation. Xenotransplantation, no matter how scientifically promising or potentially lifesaving, poses critical questions demanding a broad societal examination that considers public health; the perspectives of transplant physicians, nurses, and staff; and the needs and views of patients and their families. This chapter explores the potential impact of xenotransplantation on physicians and health care providers, individual patients, and society. Consideration is given to the value and quality of human life, special problems of informed consent, and the use of animals. The chapter also addresses issues regarding the economic and regulatory impact of xenotransplantation.

PATIENTS, ETHICS, AND SOCIETY

Patients' Perspectives

One of the most compelling parts of the workshop was a panel that included patients, family members, and advocates. The individuals on this panel discussed their experiences waiting for organs, undergoing allotransplants, or working to obtain experimental xenotransplants for others. The nature and style of the arguments in other parts of the workshop, based on scientific and philosophical reasoning, were in stark contrast to the personal stories and perceptions of those whose lives had been directly affected by diseases for which transplants or novel medical therapies offered the only hope of survival.

One of the clearest messages conveyed how patients often feel excluded from decisions made by the medical, scientific, ethical, and public policy communities. The debate about transplanting baboon bone marrow into an AIDS patient in San Francisco prominently displayed this message for two reasons. First, the experiment in question was in the process of being considered for approval by the Food and Drug Administration (FDA). Second, AIDS patient activists in favor of the experiment represent a well-organized and sophisticated patient advocacy group that has been successful in bringing patient perspectives to debates about the accessibility and applications of new AIDS therapies. A leader from this community pointedly reminded the committee that it should have included a patient representative.

Brenda L. from Project Inform in San Francisco presented the position of AIDS activists by directly addressing some of the most common conflicts among stakeholder groups. For example, regarding research into new therapies, she asked:

> What is the ultimate goal? Is it to answer questions that pertain to the public health or is it to answer interesting academic questions? Compounded with this is the fact that it is difficult to know if those interesting questions are going to impact on the public health or if they will just raise more interesting academic questions. One has to wonder if some of the delays aren't just due to pure academic rhetoric flying back and forth. One knows that a lot of delays are happening because the scientists have proprietary interests over their own science. Sometimes industry and their proprietary interests get involved. That invariably ends up hurting the patient population.

On issues of informed consent, the AIDS bone marrow experiment is unique in that the patient actively participated in much of the planning and development of the experimental procedure. Nevertheless, Ms. L. spoke about the subjects in early transplant experiments in terms with which many physicians and ethicists would likely agree.

> As with any new procedure, there will be those who will sacrifice their lives in the name of science. The history of transplantation clearly has been such that most people who participate in earlier studies don't fare as well. These first patients carried a heavier burden of risk. However, if it weren't for their participation, such as in the early lung transplants, and some of them actually sacrificing

their lives to participate in research, we would not be where we are
today with organ transplantation.

Although much in the public eye, the application of xenotransplants for
AIDS is but one potential benefit from a patient perspective. There are
thousands of people with kidney, liver, and heart disease who also face the real
possibility that lifesaving therapy will not be available to them. This view was
voiced by another member of the panel, Len K., a 38-year-old man who had
been waiting for a kidney transplant for a year and a half and had undergone
peritoneal dialysis.[1] His kidney disease, caused by severe diabetes and
hypertension, forced him to be on Social Security Disability and created
financial and health-related insecurities that seriously disrupted the lives of Len
and his wife Maryanne.

> *I am comfortable on disability . . . on the one hand, the idea of*
> *disability, in terms of my mental state, is pretty good, and I am*
> *adjusting to it well. On the other hand, when I go to a conference,*
> *or hear about people my age or people I grew up with or worked*
> *with, and I see them get promotions, advance in their careers, or*
> *have families, that gets me down . . . there has been an impact, I*
> *know, on Maryanne. With my constant illness and with a variety of*
> *major events such as triple-bypass surgery, kidney failure, arthritis,*
> *and a variety of skin diseases—mostly related to the dialysis—it*
> *takes an effect on Maryanne. I think that a lesser woman would*
> *have left me . . . given what Maryanne has put up with, I think it is*
> *amazing.*

Three other persons shared their experiences with workshop participants.
Gloria B. and Calvin W. had received organ transplants. The third person,
Evelyn W., was Calvin's mother, who spoke about the issues confronted by
families. Gloria B., a mother of two, had experienced acute liver failure due
to an extremely severe case of hepatitis A. By the time she reached the first
hospital, Gloria was near death and only occasionally conscious. Her family
was forced to make the decision to put her on artificial life support or to let
her die. However, another option became available when she was transferred
to a hospital capable of doing liver transplants and, fortunately, a liver became
available. Gloria's family agreed to the liver transplant immediately. Despite
their questions, with time running out, they felt they had to proceed.

---

[1]Len K. received a kidney transplant in January 1996. His recovery has been
complicated by a stroke following surgery.

Calvin W. also contracted hepatitis, but as an infant in 1972. For years, Calvin's mother and doctors did what they could to "patch him up" from numerous complications of the disease. In 1986, when liver transplants became available for pediatric patients, only a very few had been done. Calvin, however, was deteriorating rapidly and was given a transplant, after extensive discussions involving Calvin, his family, and his physicians. Even Calvin's doctor, however, expected that a second transplant would eventually be necessary. Getting Calvin to the second transplant was a particular challenge because a suitable donor was not available quickly. To "bridge" Calvin and buy him time, doctors offered to perform a procedure in which Calvin's blood would be perfused through a pig's liver—essentially a temporary xenotransplant. Calvin's mother, Evelyn, recalled the decision this way:

> *When they offered me the pig, I didn't think about the fact that it was a pig. I thought, "We are losing this battle, and desperate men take desperate measures." We were desperate . . . At that point Calvin could not speak for himself, and I was his proxy. As such I was going to do everything I possibly could to see him through this. If he did not want it done, then he was going to have to tell me that when this was all over.*

Both Calvin's second liver transplant and Gloria's first liver transplant have been, from a medical point of view, successful, but what about their lives afterwards? Their stories reflect those of many transplant patients in that the time following even successful transplants can be difficult for a variety of reasons. For example, Calvin's family had adequate medical insurance to cover nearly the entire cost of the transplants. Indeed, his family had been more adversely affected financially by the frequency and expense of medical care before the transplants. In contrast, Gloria B.'s family struggled for more than a year to get its health maintenance organization to pay $300,000 toward the $500,000 expense of the transplant. A large portion (the average is approximately 82 percent) of Len K.'s kidney transplant will be paid entirely by Medicare's End Stage Renal Disease Entitlement Program. For many others, no insurance or Medicare program is available, and because of lack of money, many of these patients will die.

Although economic issues loom large for transplant patients, they face other serious concerns related to quality of life and their complex reactions to the fact that another person's organ resides within their bodies. Also, lifelong immunosuppressive therapy has significant side effects, which often make it difficult for patients to take these medications as directed. Feelings expressed by patients are by no means homogeneous in this regard. According to Calvin,

I really didn't realize the value of the gift with the first transplant. Although I was worried and concerned, I think I took the donation for granted a little. Now, after the second transplant, I appreciate the donor more, including taking the medication and everything.

Gloria, however, said,

My immediate reaction was—I wouldn't say anger—probably a bit of disgust with myself mixed with confusion because the whole process was so foreign to me and I felt almost like a guinea pig, they were just doing anything to keep me alive. I wondered how important is that, because now I am going to deal with having this organ inside me that does not belong to me. Left up to me and as I didn't have any prior knowledge [about transplantation and donors], and I had some say-so in the matter, I'm not so sure I would have made the same decision for myself.

Reactions such as these are by no means unique, and they illustrate the deep complexity of patients' views about their health, their lives, and the means by which their lives are preserved. When asked, some patients embrace xenotransplantation as a wonderful answer to their prayers for a reasonable medical treatment. Others, for equally important personal reasons, reject such treatment. Despite the complexity of their reactions, one response seemed almost universal among transplant patients: they want to be heard and to participate in decisionmaking. Such decisionmaking occurs at many levels, and achieving maximal patient participation is challenging. Although AIDS activists have had a large voice in regulatory matters concerning AIDS therapies, few other patient groups have had such a voice. Many patients, who are healthy enough, are actively involved in decisionmaking with their physicians, but this partnership varies greatly from physician to physician and from patient to patient. Rarely do patients and scientists participate together in decisionmaking; indeed, each is likely to bring different vocabularies and perceptions to issues, which would require extensive translation for effective communication. Fortunately, protections that encourage, and at points require, patient–physician and patient–researcher communication exist in the form of guidelines for research with human subjects.

Informed Consent

Informed consent of research subjects is required in all clinical research conducted in the United States.[2] The overall purpose of informed consent is to give potential subjects information that will enable them to make freely chosen, knowledgeable, and careful decisions about whether they wish to participate in research. Federal regulations require that the consent form contain a description of the nature and purpose of the research and its risks, benefits, and alternatives, among other requirements (45 CFR 46). The form must be approved by the local institutional review board (IRB) before it is given by the physician/researcher to a prospective participant for his or her consideration.

At this early stage, xenotransplant research carries high risks and high uncertainties in the setting of possibly desperate patient need, a situation that places added weight on informed consent. For example, more research needs to be done on the psychological, religious, and social interpretations of xenotransplants for patients and their families. In addition, for the patient, the risks are especially great relative to the individual benefits, and for the community, there is a possible public health risk from animal pathogens or new infectious agents.

The history of organ transplantation is replete with instances of medical community enthusiasm tending to underestimate risks and exaggerate individual benefits of new medical and surgical interventions (Arnold, 1995; Fox and Swazey, 1992). Overly optimistic judgments have appeared repeatedly in public statements by treating physicians and in consent forms. In one example, the permission form signed by the parents of Baby Fae—the neonate who received a baboon heart in 1985 for treatment of a congenital defect—clearly overstated the benefits in light of what was known at the time: "Long-term survival with appropriate growth and development may be possible following heart transplantation . . . this research is an effort to provide your baby with some hope of immediate and long-term survival." Baby Fae survived four weeks, after which no whole organ xenotransplants were attempted for eight years. Given that none of the more than 20 xenotransplant patients has survived longer than 9 months, and most for considerably shorter periods, xenotransplants must be considered extremely risky. The benefits, if

---

[1]Consent is required in both publicly funded and privately funded research, through the Department of Health and Human Services (HHS) and FDA regulations, respectively. HHS regulations (45 CFR 46) allow an institutional review board to waive the requirement for informed consent in certain circumstances—for example, when the research in question involves no more than minimal risk, does not adversely impact subjects' rights and welfare, and could not be carried out without the waiver.

any, in the short term are likely to be highly limited. The patient may die immediately, may experience increased pain and suffering before dying, and/or may survive somewhat longer than otherwise. In contrast, the benefits to "society" may be significant because the new knowledge gained may benefit future patients.[3] In this kind of circumstance, when the personal benefits are likely to be disproportionately low relative to the high degree of risk, informed consent assumes even greater prominence.

The former director of the National Institutes of Health (NIH) Office of Protection from Research Risks, Charles McCarthy, has offered suggestions for the content of informed consent for xenotransplant recipients. These suggestions, which are based on criteria listed in federal regulations, include a clear statement of the early stage of the research; mortality and morbidity data from previous human recipients (including quality of life); the option of no treatment; a fair estimate of the risks and of the time that will elapse between the xenotransplant procedure and the availability of a human organ (if the xenotransplant is to serve as a "bridge"); and disclosure of the degree of media attention on patients and their families and of the likelihood of offers to "sell" their story (McCarthy, 1995).

Apart from obligations to patients, what are investigators' obligations to provide information to, or seek some form of consent from, health care workers, family members, and the public? These groups may bear a risk, however difficult to quantify, of unwitting exposure to emerging pathogens.

There is no legal requirement for informed consent of "third parties" (i.e., people who are in contact with the research subject). Third-party risks are not normally evaluated in the course of the IRB approval process, and if the IRB does approve a research project involving a human subject, neither disclosure nor the consent of third parties is required. In the absence of legal mandates, is there an ethical obligation? What follows is first a discussion of the capability of the IRB to assess third-party risks and then a discussion of disclosure and/or approval of third parties.

Some have suggested that IRBs lack formal guidance in defining and assessing third-party risks (Dresser, 1995). The only explicit guidance on third-party risks comes from the field of gene therapy. When investigators develop gene therapy protocols for review by the NIH Recombinant DNA Advisory Committee and by the FDA, they are guided by the "NIH Guidelines for Research Involving Recombinant DNA Molecules." One of the appendixes to

---

[3]The Federal Regulations for the Protection of Human Subjects (45 CFR 46) require that the degree of risk be "reasonable" in relation to the degree of benefit, either to the individual or to society (in the form of knowledge gained). The final determination of whether the benefits justify the risks is made by the IRB.

these guidelines lists the following key public health questions that investigators should address:

- On what basis are potential public health benefits or hazards postulated?
- Is there a significant possibility that the added DNA will spread from the patient to other persons or to the environment?
- What precautions will be taken against such spread (e.g., patients sharing a room, health care workers, or family members)?
- What measures will be undertaken to mitigate the risks, if any, to public health?
- In light of possible risks to offspring, including vertical transmission, will birth control measures be recommended to patients? Are such concerns applicable to health care personnel?

These are complex questions, the answers to which are fraught with unknowns. If they are addressed, another set of questions will emerge related to the content of and process for public disclosure and/or approval.

As a practical matter, obtaining informed consent of health care workers and families is much easier than obtaining informed consent from the community. Informed consent of communities is traditionally undertaken, not individually, but through public hearings, advisory bodies, and a variety of legislative and executive branch processes. Many workshop participants believed that addressing such issues for xenotransplants will require extensive discussion involving government agencies, patients and their families, and the public.

Justice and Fairness Issues:
Organ Allocation and Research

There are two major questions of justice and fairness that must be addressed in the consideration of xenotransplants: organ allocation and access to research. The United States has already developed a system for allocating human organs. The system was designed with patient and public input and with the input of physicians, ethicists, economists, and many other professionals. Despite this, support may be fragile because the scarcity is so acute that it fosters perceptions—however justified—of inequality, of organs going to the wealthiest and most powerful (Bowman, 1995).

A system for organ allocation was established by the National Organ Transplant Act (NOTA) of 1984. The system was designed to eliminate inequities in the distribution of whole organs, and the legislation created a voluntary national system of organ allocation that has operated with the support and compliance of the transplant community. This national system, the Organ Procurement and Transplantation Network, was established by the U.S. Department of Health and Human Services and is operated under contract by the Health Resources and Services Administration with the United Network for Organ Sharing (UNOS). The role of UNOS is to link all organ procurement organizations with transplant centers. It operates a national computerized waiting list of patients in need of organs, whom it matches with donors when organs become available.

The board of UNOS, in consultation with the public, set down principles for the allocation of scarce organs and created a formula for their allocation to those on the waiting list. The formula varies according to the organ, but in general it is based on medical, scientific, and ethical criteria, such as histocompatibility, blood type, waiting time, logistics, and medical urgency. The ability to pay for the transplant is not a factor in the allocation of organs to patients on the waiting list (although it does factor in elsewhere, as discussed below). When an organ becomes available, UNOS generates a list of eligible patients in priority order. If the local organ procurement organization violates the ranking or other UNOS policies, its membership may be threatened. The development of more stringent sanctions—such as the loss of Medicare and Medicaid accreditation—is in progress, based on the passage of recent federal legislation.

Inequities can occur *before* placement on the waiting list. Two critical stages precede placement on a waiting list: patients need to be referred to a transplant center, and they need to be accepted by the center (Moskop, 1991). Inability to pay factors in at both stages. Because most private and public insurance covers transplants (see section on economics below), patients who are unable to pay are either uninsured or underinsured and account for 26 percent of the U.S. population (Evans, 1989). These patients may receive medical care sporadically, if at all. If they receive care and are diagnosed adequately, they still may be less likely to be referred to a transplant center because of their inability to pay. If they are referred, the transplant center generally requires assurance of payment before placing a patient on the waiting list (Evans, 1989). Transplant centers justify this practice on the grounds that, in order to recover losses, they must charge higher rates to all patients. This barrier to transplantation, created by inability to pay, is often referred to as the "green screen." Because of this barrier, many believe that the need for organs exceeds the actual number on the waiting list, but the extent of the real demand is difficult to document.

The green screen is less likely to operate for patients needing kidneys rather than other organs.[4] Inability to pay was virtually eliminated as a factor in access to kidney dialysis and transplantation with the passage in 1972 of legislation extending Medicare benefits to patients with end stage renal disease (ESRD). These benefits are available to more than 90 percent of the U.S. population (Evans, 1989). The significance of this legislation is best demonstrated by a study that compared the composition of dialysis patients *before* and *after* the legislation's passage. It revealed that before 1973, many patients were selected on the basis of social status rather than medical suitability. Afterwards, access was greatly expanded, irrespective of income, race, gender, and education (Evans et al., 1981). For example, the percentage of African Americans in the hemodialysis population climbed from 7 to 34.9 percent, the latter figure reflecting the disproportionately high prevalence of ESRD among African Americans in the U.S. population. Likewise, African Americans represent 33.7 percent of patients waiting for kidney transplants (UNOS, 1994). Ironically, African Americans experience the longest waiting times for kidneys, once they have been placed on the waiting list. Their median number of days on the list is 74 percent greater than that of whites. This disparity is due to the greater difficulty in finding suitable tissue matches for African American patients. Although the organ donation rate among African Americans is proportional to their prevalence in the general population (12 percent), it is much lower than their prevalence in the ESRD population (UNOS, 1994). Further, although suitable tissue matches are possible between African Americans and caucasians or other ethnic groups, there is a higher probability of a match between two African Americans. Thus, the total probability of finding matches for African Americans among the general organ donor population is reduced, decreasing the number of suitable organs available.

The implications of the present system of organ allocation for xenotransplants first involve the **pressure of the organ shortage** and its effects on the search for alternatives. From the patient's perspective, there is much confusion and uncertainty about the true fairness or equity of the present system. Whether or not disparities will result in higher rates of xenotransplants among specific groups is not clear. If such a disparity occurs, further questions will have to be addressed. For example, will the disparity differentially affect specific ethnic or age groups? In part, the importance of these questions will depend on whether or not xenotransplants are (1) as successful as allotransplants and (2) equal to allotransplants in terms of expense. If the answers to

---

[4]Kidney patients' access may be hindered by other factors besides inability to pay. The role of the dialysis center in referring kidney patients for transplantation needs to be explored, because some have suggested that for-profit dialysis centers have a financial interest in keeping patients rather than referring them for transplant.

both of these questions show xenotransplants to be equal to allotransplants, possible disparities across regions or ethnic groups may not constitute a lack of fairness or equity. Such answers, however, await a long period of research and technological development.

Equitable access to research, then, is the other major concern about xenotransplants in particular. The significance of "equitable access" has changed dramatically over time. Historically, concerns centered on unequal burdens or levels of exploitation of religious groups, minorities, and the disabled (Bowman, 1995). The Nazi medical experiments and the Tuskegee syphilis study represent egregious examples of inequality and exploitation. The legal and ethical commitment to informed consent and equitable selection of research subjects evolved out of these shameful legacies. The U.S. Department of Health and Human Services Regulations for the Protection of Human Subjects attest to the preeminence of informed consent and also mandate the IRB to ensure that the "selection of subjects is equitable" (45 CFR 46).

Although specific groups of people were disproportionally harmed in research in the past, the current emphasis is that historically oppressed groups not be deprived of research participation. Research participation is seen now by many as a benefit, a possible lifesaving alternative to conventional treatments. The women's movement claims as one of its successes, for example, the passage of legislation[5] *requiring* the participation of women and minorities in clinical research on conditions that affect them. However, given the historical shifts back and forth, it is difficult to predict whether a positive perception of research by the public will persist in the future.

In light of the scarcity of organs, access to xenotransplant research is likely to be highly sought by many individuals. Researchers may be pressured by patients, families, and their advocates. The situation may become analogous to that immediately before the passage of NOTA, when some families took to the airwaves to dramatize their plight, a practice that has continued over time. More recently, when approval for one of the first xenogeneic bone marrow experiments for AIDS patients was delayed for almost two years, one of the investigators, Suzanne Ildstad, publicly reported being approached by several foreign governments to conduct the trial in their countries. Sensitivity about research is, nevertheless, still a strong motivating factor in minority communities. This distrust could easily lead to the perception that animal organs as experimental therapies will be offered to desperately sick people who lack the financial resources for allotransplants or are members of racial or ethnic minorities.

---

[5]The NIH Reauthorization Act of 1993.

Social Acceptance of Xenotransplants

It is difficult to assess how a society as pluralistic as our own will view an unusual or innovative medical technology. As the workshop made clear, there are many stakeholder groups involved in the development of xenotransplantation. These groups—including patients, physicians, scientists, public health officials, biotechnology researchers and investors, ethicists, and others—often have conflicting priorities and concerns. Will xenotransplantation rouse community fears and anxieties? Will the public demand that xenotransplantation not be undertaken because of the risk of infections or will the public by and large embrace xenotransplantation as a potentially lifesaving procedure? Will such approval be dependent on the species of animal used, (i.e., pigs instead use of baboons)? Human organ donation serves as an initial backdrop for understanding and anticipating broader societal reactions to xenotransplantation.

The public endorses human organ transplantation—at least on the surface. There is widespread public acceptance of organ donation and transplantation, as evidenced by a 1993 Gallup survey sponsored by the Partnership for Organ Donation (Spital, 1995).[6] In the survey of more than 400 adults, 85 percent expressed support for organ donation, although the level was somewhat lower for minority respondents. The survey found that people generally believe that organ donation allows something positive to emerge from a person's death and helps families to cope with their grief. Nevertheless, only 52 percent of these respondents had actually discussed their wishes to donate organs with a family member, and only 28 percent had ever formally granted permission for organ donation.

The disparity between attitudes and deeds may reflect many factors, including the relatively recent emergence of organ transplantation and the perceived conflicts with certain religious traditions regarding the body, as well as deep-rooted fears and anxieties about death, dismemberment, having living parts of another's body within oneself, and dehumanization. In addition, some persons are suspicious about the degree to which organ procurement fosters exploitation and premature harvesting of organs, although such practices clearly violate medical ethics and legal mandates. Such public unease may indicate a lack of trust in the medical profession.

The complex emotional underpinnings of organ donation may be difficult to capture or, indeed, may be concealed in public surveys. For example, each person responding to a survey could do so from a variety of viewpoints,

---

[6]The survey also found xenotransplants to enjoy less support than allotransplants, but the level of support did reach 50 percent.

including that of a patient needing a transplant, a family member of a dying potential organ donor, or a potential organ donor. For each viewpoint, multiple psychological, cultural, religious, and other factors come into play that reflect a respondent's deepest beliefs about, and concepts of, self and those concerning relations to known and unknown others. Yet, social altruism is a strong value in this society, and some argue that surveys regarding organ transplantation are overly positive due to the eagerness of respondents to affirm what is widely expressed as a public good—the saving of another life (Siminoff et al., 1995).

Recent public policies and proposals designed to foster donation may have had the unintended consequence of heightening apprehensions (Fox, 1995). For example, although at least 26 states have passed laws requiring that relatives of a dying patient be asked about donating the person's organs for transplant, the number of organs donated has not increased appreciably. Furthermore, proposals of presumed consent (the assumption that, in the absence of specific instructions to the contrary, a dying patient would consent to donation) and financial incentives for donation have not been implemented in the United States, but have been tried in Europe. The fact that the overall rate of organ donation remains about the same has led to even more aggressive steps to increase donation, such as the American Medical Association (AMA) endorsement of the use of tissue and organs from anencephalic babies in whom the brain, particularly the cerebral cortex, fails to develop normally. Within months, the AMA rescinded this endorsement (AMA, 1995; Gianelli, 1995). Some social observers express concern that such steps conflict with established criteria for organ donations and, more importantly, will diminish the dignity and value of human life. Some argue that as our society moves away from an inviolate and unique regard for human life, dignity, and death, the introduction of xenotransplantation may exacerbate the problem by blurring the boundaries between humans and animals.

Transplant surgeons and ethicists also voice concerns that exaggeration of the scientific potential of xenotransplants will actually reduce the number of human organs now being donated. They view public support for voluntary cadaveric organ donation as tenuous enough to be undermined easily. Although they share the hope that xenotransplantation can ameliorate the organ shortage, they are concerned that the "unnaturalness" of, or aversion to, xenotransplantation may erode public support for allotransplant donation. Indeed, the prospect of reliance on xenotransplants may undermine the symbolism of organ donation as an ultimate human gift. Sociologist of medicine Renee Fox stated at the workshop, "We would progressively lose what is perhaps the deepest and highest symbolic moral and existential significance of organ transplantation, its gift exchange dimension . . . that the living parts of persons are offered in life or in death to known or unknown others, to our strangers and our enemies as well as to our kin, in the form of a gift beyond duty and claim, beyond reckoning and rules" (Fox, 1995).

In contrast to these views, others argue that reliance on xenotransplants would bolster human dignity (Rothman, 1995). Alleviating the organ shortage may strengthen our respect for human life by curtailing exploitative practices of human organ procurement in some Third World countries. The prospect of a plentiful supply of organs might undercut the practice in India and some other countries of selling organs from live donors. Other practices that might be eliminated occur in China, where organs are harvested after death from prisoners *without* their consent. Such hopes, however, may not be realized if cultural values against the use of animal organs in these countries outweigh values about human life. Alternatively, if xenotransplantation requires special animal facilities and increased expenditures, economically depressed countries may continue exploitative practices to procure human organs.

A final concern is that the use of xenotransplantation may complicate, rather than solve, the organ shortage. There are limits to the availability of nonhuman primates, and there may well be limits on the availability of transgenic swine (if they prove to be a successful organ source). Regulations concerning animal testing for infectious diseases are among the factors that will dictate the feasibility and expense of producing organs from these animals. Moreover, should xenotransplants prove successful as "bridges" to human organ transplants, the shortage of human organs will continue to be a problem. In fact, the shortage may get worse as the demand likely increases. This is precisely what happened after the first successful kidney transplants in the 1960s—the organ shortage grew along with increasing medical achievements.

Social Acceptance of Infectious Disease Risk

The possibility of disease transmission from xenotransplantation and its effect on public perception of the procedure must be addressed. The literature on risk perception discussed in an earlier report by the National Research Council (1989) makes clear that public perception of risk almost always differs from expert judgment of risk. Public perceptions are influenced not only by scientific probabilities, but also by a host of psychological, social, economic, ethical, political, and other concerns.

Many of the conditions surrounding infectious disease risks from xenotransplants contribute to heightened public concern. The mere fact that the public derives no direct benefit from the procedure may tend to alter the risk–benefit equation by enhancing perceived risks. Lifesaving xenotransplants benefit the individual recipient and family, rather than society. Other features of xenotransplants likely to heighten public concern include scientific uncertainty about the likelihood of disease transmission; intense media attention to the first xenotransplants; a cultural distrust of science, particularly if industry investment is at stake (i.e., transgenic pigs, encapsulants); the esoteric nature of xenotransplantation science, which combines such specialized fields as immunology, molecular biology, and virology; the involuntary nature of exposure to disease (if the risk is airborne); and the possibility of a latent, occult illness that might not become manifest for years. More than a decade's worth of experience with the HIV (human immunodeficiency virus) pandemic is sufficient to alert the public to the sometimes delayed expression of zoonotic infection. In addition, current media interest in deadly viruses, as evident in books and movies about the monkey colony infected by Ebola virus in Virginia, has certainly captured, and possibly sensitized, public attention and concern.

There have also been periods of intense public outcry surrounding the introduction of recombinant DNA technology since the 1970s. The concerns have often centered on the possibility that a hybrid virus would escape the laboratory and infect humans. Even though the scientific community had acted earlier to impose a moratorium until safety guidelines were in place, communities remained distrustful. Citizens of Cambridge, Massachusetts, opposed to recombinant DNA research at Harvard and the Massachusetts Institute of Technology, were successful in convincing their city council to impose a moratorium on the research until a citizen review board could evaluate the problem and recommend action. The board, composed entirely of nonscientists, agreed to permit the research to proceed, provided additional public safety measures were imposed. Whether similar community response will occur with xenotransplantation remains to be seen.

Although the various measures outlined in Chapter 3 and recommended in Chapter 5 will reduce the likelihood of any harm to the public health from xenotransplantation, these measures cannot eliminate all risks. Refusal to proceed, however, to avoid any possibility of harm to public health would likely forestall benefits for those whose health or continued life depends on successful xenotransplantation research. During the workshop the point was made repeatedly that, in the simplest terms, we as a society are obliged to choose between two risks of harm: to those who will suffer from illnesses potentially treatable by xenografts versus those who might suffer from infectious diseases potentially let loose in the general population by xenotransplantation. Ensuing committee discussion and correspondence was considerable on this topic and in addressing this choice, some committee members were guided by what they regarded as the moral imperative that our own humanity is diminished if, in order to protect ourselves, we turn away from others whose suffering is both clearly visible to us and more clearly devastating in its impact on them. This viewpoint, then, further holds that we are morally obliged not only as individuals, but as a community, to accept some risk to ourselves to save our fellow human beings from more certain harm. Accordingly, and given this choice, we are also obliged to do all within our power as a society to protect the community from the possibility of infectious disease as we proceed with xenotransplantation.

VALUE AND USE OF ANIMALS

The use of animals in scientific research has been decried by some as unethical, a viewpoint that arose in the mid-eighteenth century and is held today by a number of spokespersons such as Tom Reagan and Peter Singer, philosophers, and Ingrid Newkirk, director of People for the Ethical Treatment of Animals. In fact, this viewpoint has engendered a debate that has become increasingly acrimonious in the past two decades. The following discussion of this issue begins by tracing briefly the history of philosophical and ethical thought on the use of animals in research. It then focuses specifically on the use of animals as a source of organs. The history of attitudes regarding xenotransplantation will be reviewed briefly, followed by modern-day reflections on the use of nonhuman primates and swine as a source of cells, tissues, and organs for transplantation.

Ethical Theory

René Descartes (1596–1650), the seventeenth century mathematician and philosopher, concluded that animals were automatons with the semblance of life, but without feelings or emotions. Because animals reacted only reflexively to external stimuli and did not have the capacity to suffer, humans could treat animals as they wished. Few people agree with this formulation today, primarily because it does not accord with their experience with pets and other animals. Instead, notions of stewardship toward animals, which existed before Descartes, have been more fully developed. Ethical theories have been proposed by philosophers and ethicists to formalize ideas of stewardship toward animals and to critically assess how these feelings may be applied to the use of animals by humans.

Ethicists address the general issue of what people ought to do and how they ought to behave. Moral arguments are developed and examined to determine if they can rationally support the actions and behavior of people. That is, ethicists study the question of what actions are considered good or bad and develop criteria for classifying decisions as good or bad. It is a rational approach to problem solving that relies on facts and logical inference, thereby enabling sound judgments. However, there is not yet a single, widely accepted and defensible theory that outlines rules of conduct toward all animals, whether they are used for scientific research, entertainment, food, or clothing.

Thus, at the current stage of development, ethical theories inform the present debate but do not settle it.

Two theories concerning the use of animals have been championed in the recent past: a utilitarian approach and a rights approach. For the purpose of efficient analysis, human activity can be divided into three components: the person performing the action, the action itself, and the consequences of that action. Utilitarian theory focuses on the consequences of an action and, hence, is a form of consequentalism, whereas rights theory considers the action itself. The utilitarian approach is discussed first, followed by the rights approach.

Utilitarianism was first enunciated by Jeremy Bentham (1748–1832), an English jurist and philosopher, and expanded by John Stuart Mill (1806–1873), an English philosopher and economist. A type of consequentialist or teleological theory, utilitarianism is best understood as a risk–benefit analysis in which the sum of the goods brought about by a certain action is weighed against the sum of the harms caused by that action. Originally, good was defined as pleasure and harm as pain, suffering, or decreased happiness.

This approach seems to accord with the way people often think about moral decisions, including the use of animals in research. Finding a new vaccine, such as the polio vaccine, or finding a cure for a disease far outweighs any harm that may befall the animal. This analysis, however, does not take into account the capacity of the animal to feel pleasure or happiness or to be free of pain and suffering. Peter Singer, a contemporary Australian philosopher, adds the loss of this good for the animal to the utilitarian analysis of the use of animals in research. Singer notes that much research involving animals appears to produce no useful results, and there may be an alternative that maximizes good without using animals in research. He concludes that the vast quantity of such research is not morally justified. Because utilitarian theory requires an estimation of the probability that a certain action will produce a good consequence, if most research produces no useful result, it is morally groundless or problematic. Alternatives to the use of animals in research may include conducting public health research or epidemiological studies instead of using animals. For example, if an epidemiological study shows that the incidence of heart attack drops when fat and cholesterol intake are decreased and when the individual exercises, then public education would be a way to maximize the good far more than animal research. This analysis ignores scientific questions concerning the links between myocardial infarction and cholesterol or exercise.

Two sets of criticisms of utilitarian theory include its not taking into account the worth of the individual and its defining ultimate good as hedonistic pleasure, rather than any number of other possible goods. Because some people are willing to grant sentient animals some moral status, the individual animal's interests must be considered when assessing the probable consequences of an action. This does not mean that an animal is to be accorded an equal moral status to humans or that the life of a human is equal to the life of an animal. It is clear that the quality of human life in its totality (including cognitive development and the ability to feel and discuss emotions) is far richer and more complex than the life of any animal. Thus, one should give more weight to human than to animal life. The notion of complexity of life can be extended to our intuitive ideas that the life of a nonhuman primate is worth more than that of a mouse, which in turn is more complex than a paramecium. Thus, according to Singer, a more complete utilitarian analysis would include the rights of individuals as autonomous agents and a broad definition of "the good" to encompass the complexity of life.

The second approach to ethics, the rights approach, is indebted to the philosophy of Immanuel Kant (1724–1804), a German philosopher, who stated that humans are ends in themselves and thus have certain rights. The rest of nature is viewed as existing to serve human interests; in particular, animals exist "merely as a means to an end. That end is the good of humankind." According to this formulation, humans are morally free to use animals as they wish, provided that the animals are not treated cruelly (because to do so might make humans cruel to each other). This approach views acts as right or wrong regardless of their consequences. Thus, rights or deontological theorists reject the utilitarian approach. Instead, their view is that what is right does not depend on the value of the consequence, but on appropriate treatment of the individual. Furthermore, rights theory focuses on the inherent rights of individuals, not on the sum of the interests of a group of people.

What Kant developed is what Tom Regan, a modern American philosopher, would term an extreme rights position. Regan moderates Kant's position by allowing some utilitarian concepts to enter the discussion, but he maintains that "rights are more basic than utility and independent of it." Regan argues that all individuals, including nonhuman animals (because we cannot distinguish all humans from all animals), are to be treated with respect. He then holds that nonhuman animals are of direct moral significance and that humans are morally responsible for their protection. The definition of sentience has vexed many rights philosophers, because many animals seem to possess a set of psychological characteristics such as memory, wants or desires, acting intentionally, and so forth. The issue of sentience and what beings inherently possess rights is unresolved. Many feel that the rights view can be expanded to include some idea of hierarchy, with humans deserving of more rights, and lower animals having far fewer. Elements of utilitarianism are incorporated into this version of the rights theory.

The rights ethical view accords with many people's view of animals, insofar as it explains why we should treat animals as individuals worthy of respect. Most people would agree that humans are not free to treat animals as if they were inanimate objects, because many animals do seem to possess psychological characteristics similar to humans. The rights view also undergirds several principles that have been articulated to govern the use of animals in scientific research. Thus, the U.S. Government's Principles for the Utilization and Care of Vertebrate Animals Used in Testing, Research, and Training contains the statement (Principle IV) that "proper use of animals, including the avoidance or minimization of discomfort, distress, and pain when consistent with sound scientific practices, is imperative." Because individual animals are to be treated with respect, another of the government principles states, in effect, that the fewest possible animals should be used in research and that animals are not to be killed wantonly.

Many critics of the animal rights view espouse the idea of kinship, that is, our duty or obligation to our children, family, and country and, more broadly, to the human species. This accords with personal experience and even allows for special feeling toward our pets and domestic animals. The obvious drawback of this formulation is that it seems to be exclusionary, rather than impartial or fair. Finally, several modern philosophers have noted that all of the above theories fail to recognize that humans do not operate in a vacuum, but in fact are part of the whole of nature and must act accordingly. Often called moral ecology or deep ecology, this view talks about humans' obligations to treat the whole of nature with respect. Nature is viewed not as a "renewable resources" but rather as the context in which we exist, and it must be considered as a whole or unity. These ideas, which have been applied to the treatment of animals by Strachan Donnelley, a contemporary moral philosopher from the Hastings Center, seem to have much intuitive appeal because they incorporate elements of both utilitarianism and rights philosophies and recognize the complexity of life. This approach broadens the view from the individual to a whole community, including humans and animals, and recognizes that the complexity and richness of nature are characteristics that are due respect and protection. According to this view, endangered species are due more protection than a laboratory mouse.

History of Social Responses to Xenotransplantation

Physicians have been interested in using animal tissues to treat human disease for centuries (Lederer, 1995). In the seventeenth century, transfusion of blood from animals into people was abandoned after limited use. Mid-nineteenth century experiments by the English obstetrician James Blundell, transfusing sheep blood into dogs, suggested that human-to-human transplantation would be more effective than animal-to-human transplantation. Xenografting received more attention in the late nineteenth and early twentieth centuries. There were efforts to treat kidney failure by transplanting animal (sheep, goat, and pig) kidneys into patients. Skin grafting in patients with burns or trauma was attempted using both cadaver skin and skin from a wide variety of animals; bone grafts from living dogs were also undertaken. Gonad transplants from goats and monkeys were tried as a treatment for impotence and lack of vitality. The role of antibodies and the immune system in rejection of either human or animal tissues was not recognized until the late 1940s, when modern immunological concepts began to be described. Some surgeons were encouraged by the development of immunosuppressive agents in the late 1950s and, in the early 1960s, attempted nearly 20 primate-to-human transplants of either kidneys or livers. Ultimately all of these organs were rejected or the patients died of infections that they were unable to combat due to immunosuppression. However, it should be noted that one patient, who received a chimpanzee kidney, survived nine months and died of infection, not organ failure.

The early twentieth century experiments in xenografting prompted considerable public comment and criticism. Surgeons who attempted xenotransplantation experienced intense media scrutiny and attacks from American antivivisectionists, who also criticized the short-lived enthusiasm and ambition of surgeons for new techniques. Depictions in popular magazines and films such as the 1932 movie *Island of Lost Souls*, based upon H. G. Wells' *The Island of Doctor Moreau*, and Disney Studios' cartoon *The Mad Doctor* suggest cultural unease about the dissolution of the border between animal and human and the medical hubris that produced it.

Further public reaction was engendered by Dr. Leonard Bailey's transplantation of a baboon heart into Baby Fae in 1984. Questions concerning both the scientific basis for this transplantation experiment and the ethics of research with human subjects were raised. At the time of this experiment it was known that the success of transplantation improved when there was major blood group compatibility, a compatibility that was lacking in this case. Further, this case raised issues of how to obtain adequate informed consent under life-and-death circumstances, particularly when a child is involved.

Two points that can be made regarding these survey comments include (1) the role of the media in disseminating information and in shaping the public's understanding and acceptance of new medical procedures, and (2) the public's concern for animals, which has changed not only over the past few centuries (see above), but also over the last few decades. A new social contract concerning the use of animals in xenotransplantation may have to be negotiated, the details of which will depend on the public's response to the issues.

A Moderate Ethical Perspective of Xenotransplantation

As knowledge about biology increases and the capacity to perform such things as transplanting animal organs into people improves, more attention needs to be given to the respective value of, and relationships between, animals and humans. Utilizing closeness to being human-like as a benchmark measure of value, James Walters, a contemporary philosopher, has developed ideas that grant highest moral status to those who are closest to qualities that most humans possess (Walters, 1995). These qualities connote self-consciousness and the capacity to experience the richness of life. For Walters, the idea of proximity includes potentiality for human existence, development toward that existence, and the bonding of persons with other beings.

Walter's approach enables him to value beings in terms of their proximity or likeness to persons, rather than their being members of a biological species. He thus holds that it may be more justifiable to use anencephalic infants as organ sources than to use chimpanzees. The intelligence and human-like behavior of other species are being recognized increasingly. The language capabilities of chimpanzees approximates those of two-and-a-half-year-old human children, and wolves have a well-developed social structure. So, according to Walter's analysis, these animals may have higher moral status than some humans. Finally, it is clear that humans, like other animals, are "speciesists," in that we display partiality to fellow human beings, even if some of them lack capabilities possessed by other species. However, humans are intelligent enough and powerful enough to impose their views on the whole of nature, which imposes special obligations and constraints on human actions. This consideration raises the same issues that are considered by moral ecologists (discussed earlier).

Application to Xenotransplantation

The above review shows that ethicists and philosophers, who have addressed the morality of xenotransplants, start with differing assumptions that lead them to draw different conclusions. Most people would appear to agree with the type of thinking voiced by Walters regarding the far greater value of persons over animals that lack human abilities and characteristics. Others assume that members of the human species have the' highest priority and that appropriate, humane, and judicious use of animals is justified. Many are willing to extend some idea of kinship to certain, if not all, nonhuman primates, as well as to companion animals such as dogs and cats. For these people, the use of such animals must be justified by clear and well-articulated goals. Thus, many would not be willing to use chimpanzees as a source of organs, because they are quite human-like and because they are an endangered species. Yet they would approve of the use of baboons if this were the only alternative to the death of the patient and if the transplantation had a reasonable chance of success. It almost goes without saying that if pigs could be developed as a source of organs, most people would not object because these animals are traditionally used as a source of food, are distant from humans phylogenetically, and fall much lower on the personhood scale. Thus, although no philosophical or ethical consensus has emerged, most people would favor proceeding with well-designed xenotransplantation experiments that begin with baboons, but would favor the use of swine if these animals prove to be a viable source of organs for humans. Such experiments would be subject to review by the Institutional Animal Care and Use Committee and must be performed in accord with all applicable regulations and local institutional policy (see section below on reviewing and monitoring xenotransplantation).

ECONOMIC ISSUES REGARDING XENOTRANSPLANTS

Forecasting the economic impact of xenotransplantation is difficult at the present stage of development and eventually must address both the expense of whole organ xenotransplants and the expense of cell and tissue xenotransplants, which are likely to be quite different. The section that follows provides background information about expenditures for allotransplantation in the aggregate and at the procedure level and describes the environment in which economic decisions about xenotransplantation are likely to be made. Allotransplants are quite expensive, but the scarcity of human organs has served to limit aggregate expenditures. Despite the difficulty in prediction, xenotransplantation will certainly result in increased overall expenditures simply because success will translate need into demand.

Aggregate Expenditures for Organ Transplantation

In 1994, aggregate expenditures for organ transplantation were approximately $4.1 billion (Evans, 1995b). This figure represents a small fraction of all national health care expenditures for that year, less than half a percent of a total of almost $1 trillion. The fact that annual expenditures for organ transplantation account for only a small proportion of national health care expenditures is explained by the relatively low number of transplanted and surviving patients. Were more organs available, the total expenditures would most certainly be higher. The transplant expenditures for 1994 were incurred by approximately 125,000 surviving recipients (i.e., patients who either had undergone the procedure during the year or were receiving posttransplant care for an earlier year's transplant). The expenditures were further based on billed charges (the amount a patient or third-party payer was billed by a hospital), which are usually higher than the actual insurance reimbursement (Evans, 1995b).

Managed care, discussed more thoroughly at the end of this section, is having a profound impact on reducing organ transplant expenditures. Recent estimates indicate that, because of managed care contracting for transplant services, billed charges have decreased by approximately 34 percent (Table 4-1). So, for example, if all transplant patients were associated with a managed care network in 1994, total transplant-related expenditures would have been about $3.0 billion, rather than $4.0 billion. Thus, transplant expenditures would have represented an even lower share of national health care spending. Managed care aside, the aggregate expenditures for transplantation are relatively less visible and controversial than the high per capita expenses, that is, the expense associated with an individual.

Transplant Procedure Expenses

With annual per capita patient expenditures averaging about $33,000,[7] organ transplantation is among the most costly of medical treatments. The high expense is a function of both the surgery itself and continuing care, including immunosuppressive drugs. Organ transplants—including bone marrow transplants—consistently rank in the top ten most expensive medical treatments, according to data from the Mayo Clinic. Between 1990 and 1992, liver and heart transplants were ranked in either first or second place, based on the billing data for transplant procedures (Evans, 1993). Follow-up charges ranged between $10,000 and $21,000 in 1993. Such expenses, however, vary enormously depending on the organ (or tissue) transplanted, where the procedure is performed, and the health status of the patient before transplant. For example, average annual patient expenditures in 1994 were highest for lung transplants ($118,845) and lowest for kidney transplants ($19,195), including follow-up care (Figure 4-1). Lung transplants were the least commonly performed, accounting for only about 4 of every 10,000 transplant procedures undertaken in 1993. Kidney transplants, in contrast accounted for about 60 of every 100 transplant procedures (UNOS, 1994).

---

[7]This figure refers to billed charges as opposed to network pricing, which is considerably lower ($24,500 per patient).

TABLE 4-1 Aggregate Expenditures for Transplantation Organ, 1994

Transplant	Network Pricing	Billed Charges ($ million)	Network Effect (%)
Kidney	1,703.9	1,796.4	−5
Liver	756.4	1,344.9	−78
Heart	392.3	645.2	−64
Lung	101.4	187.3	−85
Pancreas	105.7	110.3	−4
Heart–lung	11.0	20.3	−85
Total	3,070.6	4,104.3	−3

SOURCE: Roger W. Evans, Ph.D., Section of Health Services Evaluation, Mayo Clinic, Rochester, Minnesota.

Ethics and Public Policy

Charges also vary depending on where the transplant is done. Figure 4-2 depicts the hospital charge per case and expected patient survival rates for liver transplants at different hospitals. The charges ranged from a low of $97,852 to a high of $457,522, a difference of more than 300 percent, with seemingly no effect on patient survival. The patient's health status prior to transplant also has a significant effect on charges. The poorer the health status, the higher were the charges for either heart or liver transplants. Patients on life support have the highest total charges, followed by hospitalized and then homebound patients. Not surprisingly, patients on life support before the transplant have the worst outcomes, as measured by one-year survival rates (Evans, 1993).

Expenditures for Xenotransplantation

The projected economic impact of xenotransplantation is complicated by uncertainties. These include the number of procedures that could be performed, as well as animal preparation, xenotransplant procedure, and patient posttransplant expenses. Other key variables include whether the procedure is a temporary measure to an allotransplant—and thus an additive expense—or whether the procedure is a permanent xenotransplant that might ultimately reduce the patient's long-term health care expenses. Some cellular xenotransplants, such as pancreatic islet cells or encapsulated cells, may even reduce some expenses by eliminating the need for long-term immunosuppression and its associated risks.

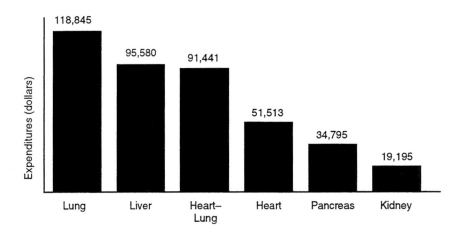

FIGURE 4-1 Average annual expenditures per surviving transplant recipient, 1994 (billed charges). SOURCE: Roger W. Evans, Ph.D., Section of Health Services Evaluation, Mayo Clinic, Rochester, Minn.

One of the greatest determinants of overall economic impact, however, is induced demand, that is, demand *created* by the availability of a procedure that is now rationed because of an inadequate organ supply. The demand will come from patients on the waiting list, patients who are not eligible for placement on the waiting list, or patients with conditions that may now benefit from xenotransplantation. It is estimated that nearly 124,000 patients, who could conceivably require a solid organ transplant, might benefit from xenotransplants. About 18,000 allotransplant procedures are now performed annually. Figure 4-3 presents an estimate of first-year expenditures with and without the availability of xenotransplants. If all those in need of a transplant receive an allo- or a xenotransplant, annual expenditures would rise from a conservative $2.9 billion to $20.3 billion, reflecting a change from less than half a percent of national health expenditures to more than 2 percent. It is important to note, however, that these estimates are quite conservative because they assume that the expense of xenotransplant procedures would be about the same as allotransplants. Further, the estimates are based strictly on the cost of the procedure (they exclude the expense associated with continuing care).

Insurance Coverage

The charges for allotransplants are covered to varying degrees by both public and private insurance, as long as the procedure is not considered experimental. Private insurers account for the bulk of the payments, with the exception of payments for kidney transplants. Kidneys are the most frequently transplanted organ, primarily because of the success of the procedure and the availability of Medicare coverage. As a result of legislation enacted in 1972, Medicare has become the primary source of kidney transplant payments, covering about 90 percent of patients (Evans, 1993).

When Congress passed the 1972 Social Security Act Amendments, Medicare was extended to cover the disabled population under age 65. At the same time, the legislation deemed patients with chronic renal failure as automatically "disabled," thus creating the first and only diagnosis-specific entitlement in the history of Medicare (IOM, 1991). Those insured under Social Security, their spouses, and dependents were thereby covered under Medicare for treatment of renal failure, including renal dialysis and transplantation. Over time, Medicare also has extended coverage to heart, liver, and bone marrow transplants, but not as an entitlement. Numerous restrictions apply. Medicaid, the joint federal–state public insurance program for certain people with low incomes, accounts for only a small proportion of organ transplants (Evans, 1993).

Private insurance usually pays for heart, liver, and bone marrow transplants, but less typically for heart, lung, and pancreas transplants, which are considered experimental by many insurers. The extent of reimbursement varies according to the policy and, as previously described, usually falls short of actual billed charges.

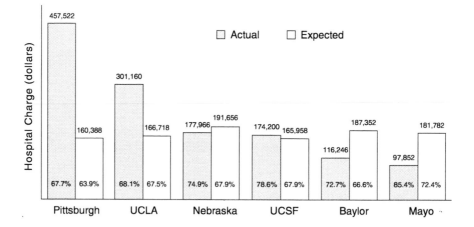

FIGURE 4-2 Liver transplantation total hospital charge per case and 3-year patient survival. SOURCE: Roger W. Evans, Ph.D., Section of Health Services Evaluation, Mayo Clinic, Rochester, Minn.

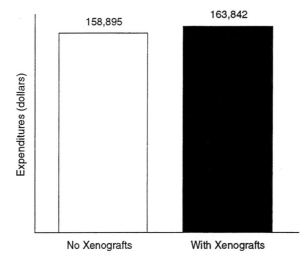

FIGURE 4-3 Impact of xenotransplantation on first-year transplantation procedure expenditures only, 1994. SOURCE: Roger W. Evans, Ph.D., Section of Health Services Evaluation, Mayo Clinic, Rochester, Minn.

Impact of Managed Care

The health care landscape is being transformed by managed care. Almost unheard of in 1980, when 3 percent of employees in medium-size and large establishments were enrolled, managed care enrollment had skyrocketed by 1993 to 49 percent of such employees (BLS, 1994).

Managed care refers mostly to health maintenance organizations (HMOs) and preferred provider organizations, which seek to provide health care in a manner that controls rising expenditures. Some of the most common cost control strategies are capitation, case management, quality reviews, and reliance on network providers who offer their services at discounted fees in exchange for a higher volume of services. Benefits typically emphasize those services that offer favorable health outcomes for the lowest expense. When two treatments are available for the same condition, managed care encourages (e.g., by offering financial incentives) or requires patients to select the least costly.

Managed care coverage of transplants is similar to that of traditional fee-for-service plans, although the data are somewhat sketchy. For example, surveys reveal that organ and tissue transplants (cornea and bone marrow) were covered by more than 90 percent of HMOs in 1992 (with the exception of heart–lung and pancreas transplants) (Evans, 1993). The major difference between managed care and fee-for-service plans is the price. Through negotiated discounts with providers, managed care organizations have succeeded at reducing transplant fees by more than one-third (Figure 4-1). Ironically, these dramatic price reductions have served to "improve" the cost-effectiveness of transplantation, although without any apparent effect on medical outcome and survival.

The introduction of any new and expensive technology into managed care is likely to encounter resistance unless it is cost-effective. Managed care providers, and the employers who contract with them and dictate many of the coverage decisions, are wary of high-expense, low-benefit technologies. For xenotransplants to be covered by managed care, their cost-effectiveness will have to be demonstrated by carefully designed studies, as was done by comparing kidney allotransplants with dialysis. Most managed care providers and other insurers have decided to cover kidney transplants because research demonstrated that annual expenditures for a patient with a functioning transplant are far lower than those for renal dialysis (Evans, 1993). The final decision about whether to reimburse or cover xenotransplantation under private insurance ultimately resides in the hands of each insurer or employer, based on a host of financial and social considerations (discussed below). Xenotransplants for healthier patients would more likely be covered because they would have greater chances for success.

Pharmaceutical company investment in xenotransplant research has also come to reflect the changing health care marketplace. Therapeutic modalities, such as encapsulated cells and tissues, that hold the possibility of a cure without the need for expensive, long-term immunosuppression are more attractive to pharmaceutical investment because of their potential cost-effectiveness. Reimbursement would be almost guaranteed if cost-effectiveness could be demonstrated unambiguously.

Justice, Fairness, and the Ability to Pay

Should society pay for xenotransplants if they are found to be successful? This is a fundamental question of justice and fairness, the branch of ethics that is concerned with questions of macroallocation and microallocation of resources and whether these decisions fairly distribute societal benefits and harms. Macroallocation refers to how society allocates resources in the broadest of terms, such as whether it pays more for health care than for defense and education; microallocation refers to how society allocates resources on a lower level, such as whether an individual HMO covers xenotransplants instead of prenatal care (Evans, 1995a,b).

If whole organ xenotransplants are as expensive as allotransplants and their success at the experimental stage induces greater demand, the previous section has demonstrated that aggregate expenses will invariably rise—by several hundred percent. If the past is any guide, Congress is likely to attempt to rein in Medicare and Medicaid expenditures, and private insurers are likely to decline coverage unless the xenotransplantation is actually cheaper than existing treatment. Should they?

The actions of Congress and private insurers are likely to reflect whether and to what extent the public is willing to pay. Congress will ask about the additional expenditures, the additional benefits (in terms of lives saved and the quality of life), whether to raise taxes to cover the expenditures, or whether to take resources from other programs. The public debates, which are likely to be no different from those surrounding other expensive health technologies, will involve compelling questions about how to quantify the benefits, including the quality and prolongation of life, increased productivity, and possible medical savings in other areas (Evans, 1993, 1995a,b). Similarly, private insurers will ask whether they must raise premiums, whether their subscribers will be willing to pay more, whether this will hurt their market position because their rates may no longer be competitive, or whether coverage of xenotransplantation should encourage them to forgo coverage of something else (Menzel, 1992, 1995). These are the kinds of questions that are exceptionally difficult to answer because they hinge on an even more fundamental, often unanswerable, question—how much is saving a life worth?

REVIEWING AND MONITORING XENOTRANSPLANTATION

Experimental protocols describing research on either patients or animals are reviewed by committees at the institution where the work is to be performed. There are many similarities in the federal regulations that govern both committees. Key among these similarities is that the regulations call for the institution to assure the Office for Protection from Research Risks (OPRR) that the committees are complying with federal regulations. Thus, the regulatory framework is a self-assurance process, with annual reporting requirements and both random and for-cause audits of the activities of the committees by OPRR. A summary of the regulations pertaining to the committee that reviews research on patients is discussed first, followed by a description of the regulations for the committee that reviews the use of animals and a consideration of reviewing complex protocols such as xenotransplantation.

The institutional review board, sometimes known as the human subjects committee, is the committee that reviews protocols that describe proposed research involving patients. Regulations governing the IRB appear in the Code of Federal Regulations (45 CFR 46). The primary aim of the IRB is to protect patients who are the subjects of a research project. The committee is composed of both female and male scientists and clinicians, at least one nonscientist, and at least one member representing the community, who is not affiliated with the institution in any way. Thus, committee membership is designed to include people with a diversity of expertise, backgrounds, and experiences. IRBs use a number of criteria in approving a research project: risks to subjects must be minimized; a risk–benefit ratio must be considered for the individual subject; selection of subjects must be equitable; informed consent must be obtained from the subject or a legally authorized representative; informed consent must be documented; safety of the subject must be ensured by the collection of appropriate monitoring data; the patient must be able to withdraw from the experiment at any time; privacy must be protected; and additional safeguards must be in place for the enrollment of prisoners, children, the mentally disabled, and others whose ability to give voluntary informed consent is uncertain or in question. Institutional officials cannot approve projects that have not been approved by the IRB. The IRB is authorized to suspend or terminate any research project. Regulations specify what must be addressed in the informed consent document. This includes full disclosure of the risks and benefits of the research, an explanation of the purpose of the research, an indication of whether medical treatment will be provided by the institution if a complication occurs, and a statement that consent is voluntary and a patient's refusal to participate in the research will not jeopardize her or his regular medical care. In addition to the regulations, OPRR issues guidelines from time to time that in practice have the force of regulations.[8] The IRB is required to maintain detailed records, which include copies of the protocol and supporting documents, minutes of all meetings, records of continuing reviews, copies of all correspondence with investigators, a membership list, and procedures followed in reviewing proposals.

The institutional animal care and use committee (IACUC) is the committee reviewing protocols for the use of animals (CFR 1–3). The overall aim of the IACUC is to promote the necessary and humane care and use of animals in research. The IACUC is composed of scientists, at least one veterinarian with expertise in laboratory animal science and medicine, at least one person who is a nonscientist, and a person who is not affiliated with the institution in any way. By regulation, the IACUC must review each proposal to use an animal in research to ensure that the protocol contains the following information: that methods described will be used to avoid or minimize pain and distress to the animal during research; that anesthetics and analgesics will be used when appropriate; that if the animal experiences severe pain or distress, it will be euthanized as promptly as possible; that animals will be well

---

[8]Guidelines have the force of regulations because the penalty for not following guidelines could be as severe as the imposition of an interdiction (i.e., OPRR could, and has, stopped an institution's ability to use federal money for research).

cared for, with veterinary care available; that all personnel must be appropriately qualified and trained; and that methods of euthanasia are in accordance with guidelines. The IACUC's powers are similar to those of the IRB: institutional officials may not approve a project that has not been approved by the IACUC; the IACUC is authorized to suspend or terminate a project if it finds that the project is not being conducted as described in the protocol; and record-keeping requirements are similar to those for the IRB. In addition, an annual report must be sent to OPRR, giving the committee membership and dates on which semiannual inspections occurred. In contrast to the IRB, the IACUC has an additional obligation to review the program for the care and use of laboratory animals at least once every six months and to inspect all areas where animals are housed or used at least once every six months.

Two aspects of both IRBs and IUCACs are drawbacks when reviewing xenotransplant protocols. First, because of the broad range of scientific areas covered by protocols presented to a committee, it is unlikely that the members of the committee can include experts in all fields relevant to each protocol. Second, the committees are not constituted to protect the public health.

Absent broad scientific expertise, the committees may be unable to evaluate the scientific basis of the investigator's proposal. According to regulations, the committees can use consultants to assist in the review, although these consultants cannot vote on the proposal. In addition, many projects are funded by agencies that are equipped to provide a peer review of the quality of the scientific basis of the proposed research. Proposals that fail to receive extramural funding may still go forward, and no attempt is made to suspend projects that do not pass external scientific review. In the case of xenotransplantation protocols, which involve questions concerning the state of current immunological knowledge, human organ availability, technical feasibility, infectious disease risks, and ethical and societal issues, the committees may be very dependent on consultants or may require national review by a committee composed of experts in the relevant fields. Further, the committees would be materially aided by federally promulgated guidelines that outlined many of the issues that committee members should consider when reviewing and monitoring xenotransplantation research. Such guidelines were being prepared for public comment by the Centers for Disease Control and Prevention, National Institutes of Health, Food and Drug Administration, and other components of the United States Public Health Service as this report was being written.

A second issue is that these committees were created to protect individual subjects or an individual animal and are not constituted to protect public health. Protection of public health must be provided by a national or international body that has both the requisite breadth of view and the required knowledge. The public health issue in xenotransplantation centers on the possibility of a transmissible infectious agent being introduced into the patient by animal organs, tissues, or cells. The potential threat to public health must be assessed, and measures to safeguard public health must be identified by properly constituted national bodies and written as a set of guidelines that the committees can use when reviewing and approving protocols.

The FDA is the agency that has the potential authority to regulate xenotransplantation. This agency, however, is accustomed to regulating manufacturers of drugs, medical devices, or biologics such as vaccines. To try to fit xenotransplantation into one of these categories may bring with it an already developed set of regulatory requirements, which might not be appropriate to the transplantation of animal organs into people. An example of a possible approach is that of recent regulations concerning human tissue banks. The need to regulate these banks grew out of the finding that tissues were a source of HIV infection for some recipients. The regulations require careful screening of the donor and extensive testing of the tissues. These regulations did not interfere with the surgical use of the tissue, relied heavily on standards already developed by the American Association of Tissue Banks, and included an important role for self-regulation. National guidelines, developed by the Public Health Service and implemented by local committees, may be a useful model for handling the potential risk to public health posed by infectious agents that may accompany the use of animal organs in xenotransplantation.

FDA Regulation of Xenotransplantation

The FDA plays a complex and evolving role in regulating human organ and tissue transplantation. This section describes FDA's current regulatory framework, which generally treats processed cells and tissues—of either allogeneic or xenogeneic origin—as biological products (FDA, 1993; Kessler et al., 1993). Given the pace and scope of innovation in the field, FDA and other federal agencies are building on this framework by developing guidelines for xenotransplantation, the subject of the second part of this section.

Current Regulatory Framework

The FDA's most stringent form of regulatory control—the requirement for premarket approval for safety and effectiveness—does not apply to whole organs, regardless of whether they are allogeneic or xenogeneic (Merrill, 1995). Organ transplantation is considered a surgical procedure conducted in the practice of medicine, an area historically outside the purview of FDA. Likewise, FDA does not require premarket approval of cells and tissues that are unmanipulated. However, the agency does require premarket approval of cells and tissues if they are pretreated or manipulated. The cells and tissues can be of allogeneic, xenogeneic, or autologous (i.e., self) origin. FDA's overall regulatory framework and the critical role of tissue processing are presented in Table 4-2. (Although this table provides a general approach, it must be understood that clinical research protocols submitted to FDA are evaluated on a case-by-case basis.)

Manipulated cells and tissues are defined, for regulatory purposes, as undergoing propagation, expansion, selection, encapsulation, or other pharmacological treatment outside the body (*ex vivo*) (FDA, 1993). Any of these methods for *ex vivo* processing of cells and tissues are viewed by FDA as meeting the statutory definition of a biological product: "any virus, therapeutic serum, toxin, antitoxin, vaccine, blood, blood component or derivative . . . applicable to the prevention, treatment, or cure of diseases or injuries of man" (Section 351(a) of the Public Health Service Act). Consequently, FDA requires manipulated cells and tissue transplants to undergo the same premarket approval requirements as other biological products. Some, however, dispute FDA's regulatory jurisdiction over manipulated cells and tissues. They argue that these do not meet the statutory definition of biological products and therefore ought not be subject to premarket approval and other legal requirements.

FDA's distinction between manipulated and unmanipulated tissues is best illustrated by bone marrow transplants. Conventional bone marrow transplants, of either allo- or xenogeneic origin, are not subject to premarket approval. However, bone marrow purged of T-cells is considered under the current regulatory framework to be manipulated. Premarket approval is therefore required. If the transplanted cells or tissues are nonliving, the regulatory approach is different. Table 4-2 shows that nonliving tissues and organs, such as pig heart valves and artificial hearts, are regulated as devices. Pig heart valves, commonly used in medical practice, are nonliving because they are pretreated with glutaraldehyde, which sterilizes the tissue and cross-links the DNA, but does not interfere with the valve's mechanical properties.

For combination products—such as encapsulated porcine islet cells—the primary mode of action dictates how the product is regulated. Although the encapsulant is considered a device, the primary mode of action is through replacement cell therapy. This means that encapsulated islets are evaluated as biological products by FDA's Center for Biologics Evaluation and Research, but input is sought about the encapsulant from medical device reviewers within another center of the agency.

What are the requirements for premarket approval of biological products? The process begins with the submission of an investigational new drug application (IND), an application for human clinical testing. The title is a misnomer for biologicals, including most xenotherapies, but it stems from federal regulations that apply identical requirements for drugs and biologicals. The IND compiles all known pharmacological and toxicological information about the product, describes the general objectives of the research, and describes a specific protocol for early safety testing in humans, called a Phase I study.[9] Several INDs already have been granted by the FDA for xenotherapies, but their content is proprietary. Because Phase I studies are designed to test for safety in a few human subjects, elaborate and expensive requirements (e.g., for "good manufacturing practices") do not apply. This has been a point of confusion with academic investigators, who erroneously think that the IND for Phase I testing in humans entails prohibitive expenditures. If the Phase I study is successful, investigators can seek FDA's approval to proceed with further clinical testing in humans in Phase II and Phase III studies—the prelude to formal licensing of the biological product. Far more stringent and expensive requirements pertain to these phases of human testing.

Genetic modifications to xenogeneic organs, tissues, and cells not only require premarket approval by the FDA but also are likely to require review by the NIH Recombinant DNA Advisory Committee (RAC). The latter body has oversight over gene therapy protocols that receive federal funding or are performed at institutions receiving federal funding. The FDA review is, by law, restricted to product safety and efficacy, whereas the RAC's review is much broader, delving into social and ethical concerns. The two reviews can proceed simultaneously.

---

[9]The IND also can be submitted for phases II and III in the same submission.

TABLE 4-1 Current FDA Regulation of Organs, Tissues, and Cells

Source	Unmanipulated			Manipulated					Nonliving	
	Allo organs	Allo cells/tissues	Xeno organs	Allo cells/tissues	Auto cells/tissues	Encapsulated cells/tissues	Transgenic cells/tissues	Antibody-treated cells/tissues	Pig heart valve	Artificial heart
Premarket approval	None[a]	None[a]	None[a]	Biologic	Biologic	Biologic	Biologic	Biologic	Device[b]	Device

[a]Infectious disease and other requirements apply, but there is no requirement for premarket approval. Xenogeneic organs may be subject to Section 361 of the Public Health Service Act, according to proposals. This section provides authority to issue regulations to control communicable diseases.

[b]Pretreated with glutaraldehyde or another agent that sterilizes or "fixes" the tissue.

SOURCE: FDA (1993) and Kessler et al. (1993).

5

Conclusions and Recommendations

The following conclusions and recommendations are based on workshop presentations and discussions, as well as review of relevant materials and extensive discussions among the committee. This chapter presents those conclusions and recommendations along with the key points that underlie them, but it does not duplicate in detail material presented in previous chapters of this report.

The progress of basic science in the field of xenotransplantation has been rapid, and clinical trials of specific applications of xenotransplantation are under way. Xenotransplantation may also be valuable for the treatment of human diseases. However, it is well recognized that infectious agents can be transmitted from animals to humans and that organisms benign in one species can be fatal when introduced into other species. Further, it is known that the pathogenicity of infectious organisms can change under a variety of conditions and that the effects of infection by some organisms, such as the human immunodeficiency virus, are delayed for years or even decades. Because xenotransplants involve the direct insertion of potentially infected cells, tissues, or organs into humans, there is every reason to believe that the potential for transmission of infectious agents (some of which may not even now be recognized) from animals to human transplant recipients is real. If established in the recipient, the potential for transmission to caregivers, family, and the population at large must be considered a real threat. **The committee concludes that, although the degree of risk cannot be quantified, it is unequivocally greater than zero.**

The committee discussed various alternatives for oversight or regulation of clinical trials in light of the risk of transmission of infectious agents to the general population by xenotransplantation. There was strong feeling among a number of committee members that special regulation of xenotransplant research is not justified because other types of research, including allotransplantation, also involve substantial risks. Other members of the committee argued that the potential for transmission of new infections to humans is a unique risk, justifying special regulations. However, all members of the committee agreed that some mechanism is needed to ensure attention to and reduction of the risk of infectious disease transmission. One mechanism acceptable to all committee members was the establishment of national guidelines. The committee was aware of and commends the efforts of the Food and Drug Administration (FDA) and the Centers for Disease Control and Prevention (CDC) in developing the first set of guidelines, which are soon to be released, but were not final before this report was complete. The development of these guidelines involved discussions with other federal agencies and representatives from stakeholder groups. The importance of such guidelines should be emphasized. Hence:

> **Recommendation 1: The committee recommends that guidelines for human trials of xenotransplantation address four major areas: (1) procedures to screen source animals for the presence of infectious organisms and consideration of the development of specific pathogen-free animals for use in xenotransplants; (2) continued surveillance throughout their lifetimes of patients and periodic surveillance of their contacts (families, health care workers, and others) for evidence of infectious diseases; (3) establishment of tissue banks containing tissue and blood samples from source animals and patients; and (4) establishment of national and local registries of patients receiving xenotransplants. Special efforts should be made to coordinate with international registries and databases.**

These areas were discussed at the workshop as key elements for the effective monitoring of infectious disease transmission. For example, screening of source animals should focus first on those organisms known to infect that animal species and known to be pathogenic in humans. However, screening broadly for a wide range of organisms should be performed while conducting early trials until evidence is provided that screening for a particular organism is unnecessary. Screening of donor tissue must be complemented with mandatory active surveillance of patients receiving xenotransplants, as well as their contacts, for the sole purpose of determining the safety of xenotransplantation. Such surveillance will require collection of tissue and serum samples and coordination of information in a central database or registry. The requirement of lifelong surveillance certainly raises dangers from potential needs for enforcement and limitation of individual freedom. Thus, individual information should be strictly confidential and should not be used to screen patients for any diseases not directly caused by xenotransplants. A collection of animal donor tissue and serum samples should also be archived to allow later testing if new or unusual infectious diseases are identified in xenotransplant recipients. Special efforts should be made to coordinate the development of a national database or patient registry with efforts already under way internationally. For example, the International Islet Registry in Germany contains information on patients who have received xenotransplants of pancreatic islet cells. Cooperative links with such registries may constitute a valuable resource for surveillance and research.

Guidelines, however, do not carry the full weight of law and, thus, can function only as one part of effective oversight of individual clinical trials. There was much discussion among committee members about the role of local institutional review boards (IRBs) and their capacity to address the multiple issues related to xenotransplantation. A requirement that individual trials be approved by a national committee, analogous to the Recombinant DNA Advisory Committee (RAC), was considered unacceptable by a number of committee members. The entire committee agreed that IRBs could, with specific augmentation and required adherence to national guidelines, provide the appropriate consideration of individual clinical trial protocols. Therefore:

> **Recommendation 2: The committee recommends that adherence to specific national guidelines be required of all experimenters and institutions that undertake xenotransplantation trials in humans. Local institutional review boards and animal care committees, in consultation with outside experts, are appropriate vehicles for review of proposed protocols, provided that they are required to conform to the national guidelines for minimizing and for continued surveillance of infectious risks.**

The committee is well aware that placing the authority for the approval of xenotransplantation trials within local IRBs and IACUCs will require an increase in, or augmentation of, the existing capacity of some of these groups. For example, conformity to the national guidelines may require expert outside advice from physicians, infectious disease experts, and veterinarians trained in microbiological screening. Ensuring appropriate surveillance procedures, including tissue banking and data filing in patient registries, may also require a local IRB to consult with outside experts. In addition, IRBs will require input from patients and their families.

Transplantation of animal organs also raises new ethical and social questions. To assist local IRBs, IACUCs, and society at large to address new ethical and social questions:

Recommendation 3: The committee recommends further investigation into the special ethical issues that are raised by xenotransplantation, particularly those related to informed consent in light of the requirement for lifetime surveillance of patients and those related to fairness and justice in allocating organs, as well as research into the psychological and social impact of receiving animal organs on recipients, their families, and members of the society as a whole.

Addressing the multiple areas that require attention, however, will necessitate ongoing review and the cooperation of federal agencies, universities, and the private sector. One mechanism could be the establishment of an advisory committee comprised of representatives of federal agencies and other relevant groups, such as basic and clinical researchers, ethicists, lawyers, and private industry. It also would be important to include patient groups and the public. An advisory committee could be charged to coordinate, *but not to regulate*, research in xenotransplantation. Rather, the mandatory adherence to the soon to be released FDA and CDC guidelines would provide the needed safeguards at the local IRB level, which could be overseen by the advisory committee without establishing a complex and, possibly costly, new regulatory structure. In addition, the advisory committee could regularly review and advise the Department of Health and Human Services on guidelines in the light of evolving knowledge. Coordination within a single federal agency is difficult because the establishment of guidelines for xenotransplants involves addressing a broad range of questions of science, ethics, and public policy currently addressed handled a number of agencies. For example, federal agencies that address the basic and clinical science of xenotransplantation and infectious disease include the FDA, the NIH, the CDC, and certain components of the Department of Agriculture, but the duties of each of these agencies do not often overlap. Monitoring adherence of local IRBs and IACUCs to national regulations, and possibly to the guidelines proposed here, is the responsibility of the Office for Protection from Research Risks. Coordination will also be required between the proposed national patient registry and the archival collection sites for patient and animal donor tissue and serum samples. Given the evolving nature of this field, tracking of research progress is required so that guidelines can be amended as new data emerge. Also, developments in other public or private sector areas, such as the establishment of specific-pathogen-free breeding colonies and advances in genetic manipulation of animal cells, will have to be considered in a broad context that includes the clinical, scientific, ethical, and social implications of new discoveries and developments. An advisory committee could also be the focal point for initiating international cooperative agreements in order to share data resources from ongoing clinical trials involving xenotransplants. To deal with these considerations:

> **Recommendation 4: The committee recommends that a mechanism be established within the Department of Health and Human Services to ensure needed coordination of the federal agencies and other entities involved in development, oversight, and evaluation of established guidelines.**

At least one scientist who participated in the workshop believed that the risk of infectious disease transmission is high enough to preclude any further human xenotransplantation trials. After considerable discussion of this view and consideration of the issues listed above that will be required to assess the risk of infection, the committee concluded that the potential benefits of xenotransplants are great enough to justify this risk. Hence:

> **Recommendation 5: The committee recommends that, when the science base for specific types of xenotransplants is judged sufficient and the appropriate safeguards are in place, well-chosen human xenotransplantation trials using animal cells, tissues, and organs would be justified and should proceed.**

Clinical trials with cellular xenotransplants are already under way, and a real danger exists that the commercial applications of xenotransplant technology will outstrip both the research base and the national capacity to address special issues raised by xenotransplantation, including the risk of disease transmission. The committee considered the total expense associated with research and technology development, especially in light of current fiscal restraints. Substantial, stable resources are needed to support research, such as virus discovery, better understanding of the physiology of transplanted organs, and mechanisms of rejection; to perform diverse, well-designed clinical trials; and to maintain patient registries, tissue and serum sample collections, and surveillance for disease in patient populations. **The committee concludes that the potential of xenotransplantation is great enough to justify funding, by federal agencies, private industry, and other sources, of research and other programs (e.g., tissue banks and patient registries) necessary to minimize the risk of disease transmission.**

References

Allan, J.S. 1995a. Presentation to the IOM Conference on Xenograft Transplantation: Science, Ethics, and Public Policy. June 25–27.

Allan, J.S. 1995b. Xenograft transplantation and the infectious disease conundrum. *ILAR J.* 37(1):37–48.

American Medical Association (AMA), Council on Ethical and Judicial Affairs. 1995. The use of anencephalic neonates as organ donors. *JAMA* 273:1614–1618.

Arnold, R. 1995. Presentation to the IOM Conference on Xenograft Transplantation: Science, Ethics, and Public Policy. June 25–27.

Bach, Fritz H., Simon C. Robson, Christiane Ferran, Hans Winkler, Maria T. Millan, Karl M. Tuhlmeier, Bernard Vanhove, Martin L. Blakely, William J. Van der Werf, Erhard Hofer, Rainer de Martin, and Wayne M. Hancock. 1994. Endothelial cell activation and thromboregulation during xenograft rejection. *Immunol. Rev.* 141:5–30.

Bach, Fritz H., Simon C. Robson, Hans Winkler, Christiane Ferran, Karl Stuhlmeier, Christopher Wrighton, and Wayne W. Hancock. 1995. Barriers to xenotransplantation. *Nature Med.* 1:869–873.

Bach, F.H., M.A. Turman, G.M. Vercellotti, J.L. Platt, and A.P. Dalmasso. 1991. Accommodation: A working paradigm for progressing toward discordant xenografting. *Transplant. Proc.* 23:205–208.

Bevilacqua, M.P., J.S. Pober, G.R. Majeau, R.S. Cotran, and M.A. Gimbrone, Jr. 1984. Interleukin 1 (IL-1) induces biosynthesis and cell surface expression of procoagulant activity in human vascular endothelial cells. *J. Exp. Med.* 160:618–623.

Bowman, J.E. 1995. Presentation to the IOM Conference on Xenograft Transplantation: Science, Ethics, and Public Policy. June 25-27.

Caplan, A.L. 1992. Is xenografting morally wrong? *Transplant. Proc.* 24(2):722–727.

Chapman, L.E. 1995. Presentation to the IOM Conference on Xenograft Transplantation: Science, Ethics, and Public Policy. June 25-27.

Chapman, L.E., T.M. Folks, D.R. Salomon, A.P. Patterson, T.E. Eggerman, and P.D. Noguchi. 1995. Xenotransplantation and xenogeneic infections. *N. Engl. J. Med.* 333(22):1498–1501.

Cooper, D.K.C. 1995. Presentation to the IOM Conference on Xenograft Transplantation: Science, Ethics, and Public Policy. June 25-27.

Cooper, D.K.C., E. Koren, and R. Oriol. 1994. Oligosaccharides and discordant xenotransplantation. *Immunol. Rev.* 141:31–58.

Dalmasso, A.P., G.M. Vercellotti, J.L. Platt, and F.H. Bach. 1991. Inhibition of complement-mediated endothelial cell cytotoxicity by decay-accelerating factor. Potential for prevention of xenograft hyperacute rejection. *Transplantation* 52:530–533.

Dresser, R. 1995. Presentation to the IOM Conference on Xenograft Transplantation: Science, Ethics, and Public Policy. June 25-27.

Evans, R.W. 1989. Money matters: Should ability to pay ever be a consideration in gaining access to transplantation? *Transplant. Proc.* 21:3419–3423.

Evans, R.W. 1993. Organ transplantation and the inevitable debate as to what constitutes a basic health care benefit. Pp. 359–391 in P.I. Terasaki and J.M. Cecka (Eds.), Clinical Transplantation 1993. Los Angeles: UCLA Tissue Typing Laboratory, UCLA School of Medicine.

Evans, R.W. 1995a. Liver transplantation in a managed care environment. *Liver Trans. Surg.* 1:61–75.

Evans, R.W. 1995b. Presentation to the IOM Conference on Xenograft Transplantation: Science, Ethics, and Public Policy. June 25–27.

Evans, R.W., C.R. Blagg, and F. Bryan. 1981. Implications for health care policy: A social and demographic profile of hemodialysis patients in the U.S. *JAMA* 245:487–491.

Faustman, D. 1995. Strategy for successful xenograft survival: Designer modification of cells, tissues and organs. Presentation to the IOM Conference on Xenograft Transplantation: Science, Ethics, and Public Policy. June 25–27.

Faustman, D., and C. Coe. 1991. Prevention of xenograft rejection by masking donor HLA class 1 antigens. Science 252:1700–1702.

Fodor, W.L., B.L. Williams, L.A. Matis, et al. Expression of a functional human complement inhibitor in a transgenic pig as a model for the prevention of xenogeneic hyperacute organ rejection. *Proc. Natl. Acad. Sci. USA* 91:11153–11157.

Fox, R.C. 1995. Presentation to the IOM Conference on Xenograft Transplantation: Science, Ethics, and Public Policy. June 25–27.

Fox, R.C., and J.P. Swazey. 1992. Spare Parts: Organ Replacement in American Society. New York: Oxford University Press.

Gaines, B.A., and Suzanne T. Ildstad. 1995. Xenoreactivity, chimerism, and tolerance. Pp. 172–188 in Suzanne T. Ildstad (Ed.), Chimerism and Tolerance. R.G. Lanes Company Publishers.

Gianelli, D.M. 1995. Ethics council reverses stand on anencephalic organ donors. *Am. Med. News* 38(48):3–8.

Hammer, C. 1989. Evolutionary considerations in xenotransplantation. Pp. 115–123 in Mark A. Hardy (Ed.), Xenograft, Vol. 25. Congress Series 880.

Hancock, W.W. 1984. Analysis of intragraft effector mechanisms associated with human renal allograft rejection: Immunohistological studies using monoclonal antibodies. *Immunol. Rev.* 77:61–84.

Ildstad, S. 1995. Presentation to the IOM Conference on Xenograft Transplantation: Science, Ethics, and Public Policy. June 25–27.

Institute of Medicine (IOM). 1991. Kidney Failure and the Federal Government. Washington, DC: National Academy Press.

Institute of Medicine (IOM). 1992. Emerging Infections: Microbial Threats to Health in the United States. Washington DC: National Academy Press.

Kahan B.D. 1995. Presentation to the IOM Conference on Xenograft Transplantation: Science, Ethics, and Public Policy. June 25–27.

Kahan, B.D., and R. Ghobrial. 1994. Immunosuppressive agents. *Surg. Clin. North Am.* 74:1029–1054.

Kaufman, C.L., Y.L. Colson, S.M. Wren, et al. 1994. Phenotypic characterizations of a novel bone marrow-derived cell that facilitates engraftment of allogeneic bone marrow stem cells. *Blood* 84(8):2436–2445.

Kaufman, C., Barbara A. Gaines, and Suzanne T. Ildstad. 1995. Xenotransplantation. *Ann. Rev. Immunol.* 13:339–367.

Keeling, M. 1995. Presentation to the IOM Conference on Xenograft Transplantation: Science, Ethics, and Public Policy. June 25–27.

Kessler, D.A., J.P. Siegel, P.D. Noguchi, et al. 1993. Regulation of somatic cell therapy and gene therapy by the Food and Drug Administration. *N. Engl. J. Med.* 329:1169–1173.

Khabbaz, R.F., W. Heneine, J.R. George, et al. 1994. Brief report: Infection of a laboratory worker with simian immunodeficiency virus. *N. Engl. J. Med.* 330:172–177.

Koller, B. 1995. Presentation to the IOM Conference on Xenograft Transplantation: Science, Ethics, and Public Policy. June 25–27.

Lederer, S. 1995. Presentation to the IOM Conference on Xenograft Transplantation: Science, Ethics, and Public Policy. June 25–27.

McCarthy, C.R. 1995. Ethical aspects of animal to human xenografts. *ILAR J.* 37(1):3–8.

McKenzie, J.F.C., S. Cohney, H.A. Vaughan, N. Osman, J. Atkin, E. Elliott, W.L. Fodor, M.A. Gallop, K.R. Oldenburg, D. Burton, and M.S. Sandrin. 1995. Overcoming the anti-Gala(1–3)Gal reaction in xenotransplantation. *Xenotransplantation* 3:86–89.

Menzel, P.T. 1988. Some ethical costs of rationing. Pp. 155–164 in Deborah Mattheiu (Ed.), Organ Substitution Technology. Boulder, CO: Westview Press.

Menzel, P.T. 1992. Scarce dollars for saving lives: The case of heart and liver transplants. *Law, Med., and Health Care* 20:57–66.

Menzel, P.T. 1995. Presentation to the IOM Conference on Xenograft Transplantation: Science, Ethics, and Public Policy. June 25–27.

Merrill, R.A. 1995. Presentation to the IOM Conference on Xenograft Transplantation: Science, Ethics, and Public Policy. June 25–27.

Michaels, M. 1995. Presentation to the IOM Conference on Xenograft Transplantation: Science, Ethics, and Public Policy. June 25–27.

Michaels, M.G., and R.L. Simmons. 1994. Xenotransplant-associated zoonoses. Strategies for Prevention. *Transplantation* 57:1–7.

Morse, S. 1995. Presentation to the IOM Conference on Xenograft Transplantation: Science, Ethics, and Public Policy. June 25–27.

Moskop, J.C. 1991. Ability to pay and access to transplantation. Pp. 433–436 in W. Land and J.G. Dossetor (Eds.), Organ Replacement Therapy: Ethics, Justice, Commerce. Berlin: Springer-Verlag.

National Research Council. 1989. Improving Risk Perception and Communication. Washington, DC: National Academy Press.

Persing, D. 1995. Presentation to the IOM Conference on Xenograft Transplantation: Science, Ethics, and Public Policy. June 25–27.

Platt, J.L. 1994. A perspective on xenograft rejection and accommodation. Pp. 127–149 in Goran Moller (Ed.), Immunological Reviews, Vol. 141.

Platt, J.L. 1995. Presentation to the IOM Conference on Xenograft Transplantation: Science, Ethics, and Public Policy. June 25–27.

Platt, J.L., G.M. Vercellotti, B. Lindman, T.R. Oegema, Jr., F.H. Bach, and A.P. Dalmasso. 1990. Release of heparan sulfate from endothelial cells: Implications for pathogenesis of hyperacute rejection. *J. Exp. Med.* 171: 1363–368.

Pober, J.S., and M.A. Gimbrone, Jr. 1982. Expression of Ia-like antigens by human vascular endothelial cells is inducible in vitro: Demonstration by monoclonal antibody binding and immunoprecipitation. *Proc. Natl. Acad. Sci. USA* 53:1851–1854.

Ricordi, C. 1995. Presentation to the IOM Conference on Xenograft Transplantation: Science, Ethics, and Public Policy, June 25–27, 1995.

Rothman, D. 1995. Presentation to the IOM Conference on Xenograft Transplantation: Science, Ethics, and Public Policy. June 25–27.

Scharp, D., C.J. Swanson, B.J. Olack, et al. 1994. Protection of encapsulated human islets implanted without immunosuppression in patients with type I or type II diabetes and in nondiabetic control subjects. *Diabetes* 43:1167–1170.

Siminoff, L., R.M. Arnold, A.L. Caplan, B.A. Virnig, and D.L. Seltzer. 1995. Public policy governing organ and tissue procurement in the United States. *Ann. Intern. Med.* 123:10–17.

Spital, A. 1995. Mandated choice: A plan to increase public commitment to organ donation. *JAMA* 273(6):504–506.

Squinto, S., and W.L. Fodor. 1995. Transgenic swine engineered to be resistant to the humoral immune system of primates. Presentation to the IOM Conference on Xenograft Transplantation: Science, Ethics, and Public Policy. June 25–27.

Starzl, T.E. 1995. Presentation to the IOM Conference on Xenograft Transplantation: Science, Ethics, and Public Policy. June 25–27. Starzl, T.E., A.J Demetris, M. Trucco, et al. 1993. Cell migration and chimerism after whole-organ transplantation: The basis of graft acceptance. *Hepatology* 17(6):1127–1152.

Swindle, M. 1995. Presentation to the IOM Conference on Xenograft Transplantation: Science, Ethics, and Public Policy. June 25–27.

Terasaki, P.I., J.M. Cecka, D.W. Gjertson, and S. Takemoto. 1995. High survival rates of kidney transplants from spousal and living unrelated donors. *N. Engl. J. Med.* 333(6):333–336.

United Network for Organ Sharing (UNOS). 1994. Annual Report of the U.S. Scientific Registry of Transplant Recipients and the Organ Procurement and Transplantation Network—Transplant Data: 1988–1994. Richmond, VA: UNOS.

U.S. Bureau of Labor Statistics (BLS). 1994. Employee Benefits in Medium and Large Private Establishments, 1993. Bulletin 2456. Washington, D.C.: U.S. Department of Labor.

U.S. Food and Drug Administration (FDA). 1993. Application of current
    statutory authorities to human somatic cell therapy products and gene
    therapy products. Federal Register Notice, October 14.
Walters, J. 1995. Presentation to the IOM Conference on Xenograft Trans-
    plantation: Science, Ethics, and Public Policy. June 25–27.

A

Workshop Agenda

XENOGRAFT TRANSPLANTATION: SCIENCE, ETHICS, AND PUBLIC POLICY

June 25–27, 1995
Bethesda Hyatt Regency Hotel—Crystal Ballroom
1 Bethesda Metro Center, Bethesda, Maryland

<u>Sunday, June 25</u>

9:30 a.m.   Welcome and Introduction
Kenneth I. Shine, IOM President
Karen Hein, IOM Executive Officer
Norman Levinsky, Committee Chair

Session I: Assessing the Science Base

9:45   Moderator's overview of session
Keith Reemtsma

10:00   Immunology: The Early Responses
Jeffrey Platt

10:15   Immunology: The Long-Term Responses
Thomas Starzl

10:30   Issues
Olga Jonasson

10:45   Discussion

11:00   Potential Therapeutic Approaches
Moderator: *Denise Faustman*

Genetic Engineering Overview
Denise Faustman

11:15   Transgenic and Knockout
               Beverly Koller

11:30   Transgenic Pigs
               Steven Squinto

11:45   Discussion

12:15 p.m.   LUNCH BREAK

1:00   Recipient Modification
               Cellular Modification/Chimerism
               Suzanne Ildstad

1:15   Nonmodification
               Camillo Ricordi

1:30   Immunosuppression
               Barry Kahan

1:45   Respondents and Discussion
               David K.C. Cooper
               Ali Naji

2:15   Panel Status of Human Trials
               Moderator: *Nancy Ascher*

               David L. Cooper
               Keith Reemtsma
               David Sharp

2:45   Discussion

3:00   BREAK

Session II: Infectious Issues—Moderator: *Stephen Morse*

3:15   Overview
                Frederick Murphy

3:45   Emerging Pathogens
                Stephen Morse

4:00   Discussion

4:20   Risk Assessment
                Jonathan Richmond

4:30   Infectious Risk and Risk Assessment
                Jonathan Allan
                Jay A. Fishman

4:50   Discussion

5:15   Adjourn

Monday, June 26

8:30 a.m.   Specific Pathogen-Free Environments and
                Nonhuman Primates
                Michale Keeling

8:40   Specific Pathogen-Free Environments and Swine
                Michael Swindle

8:50   Panel Discussion
                (*all speakers*)

10:15   BREAK

10:30   Applications to Humans
                Moderator: *Marian Michaels*

11:00   Surveillance and Public Health
                Louisa Chapman

11:30   Detection Methods
                             David Persing

12:00   LUNCH BREAK

1:00 p.m.   Panel Discussion (*all speakers*)
                             Respondents: *Jonathan Allan, Steven Deeks*

Session III: Ethics and Public Policy

Moderator: *Harold Vanderpool*

2:00   Social and Political Issues
                             Moderator: *David Rothman*

                             Addressing Questions Raised by Xenograft
                             Transplantation
                             Renee Fox

                             Commentary and Response
                             David Rothman
                             Stuart Youngner

2:45   Discussion

3:15   BREAK

3:30   Economics and Allocation of Organs and Tissues

                             Economic Impact of Xenograft Transplantation:
                             Lessons from Heart Transplantation
                             Roger Evans

3:50   Macroeconomic Aspects of Xenograft
                             Transplantation
                             Paul Menzel

4:10   Who Gets Which Organs? Questions of Justice
                             James Bowman

4:30   Discussion

4:45	Clinical Trials Panel Discussion Moderator: *Clive Callender* *Robert Arnold* *James Bowman* *Rebecca Dresser* *Stuart Youngner*
5:30	Discussion
5:45	Adjourn

Tuesday, June 27

8:30 a.m.	Value and Use of Animals Panel Moderator: *Ralph Dell* *Susan Lederer* *Justin Leiber* *Andrew Rowan* *James Walters*
9:30	Discussion
9:45	Issues for Regulatory Review Moderator: *Robert Burt* *Richard Merrill*
10:15	Discussion
10:30	BREAK
10:45	The Patients' Views Panel Moderator: *John Robinson* (counselor) *Gloria B.* Liver transplant patient *Brenda L.* Project Inform *Calvin W.* Multiple transplant patient, and his mother, Evelyn W. *Len K.* Potential kidney transplant patient

11:45   Discussion

12:15 p.m.   Wrap-Up
                         Norman Levinsky and *Session Chairs*

12:45   Adjourn

SPEAKERS AND PANELISTS

Jonathan Allan, D.V.M.
Southwest Foundation for Biomedical
  Research
Department of Virology and
  Immunology
San Antonio, TX

Robert Arnold, M.D.
Associate Professor of Medicine
University of Pittsburgh School
  of Medicine
Pittsburgh, PA

James Bowman, M.D.
Professor Emeritus
Department of Pathology, Medicine,
  and Committee on Genetics
University of Chicago
Chicago, IL

Gloria Brooks
Fort Washington, MD

Louisa Chapman, M.D.
Medical Epidemiologist
National Center for Infectious
  Diseases
Centers for Disease Control
  and Prevention
Atlanta, GA

David K.C. Cooper, M.D., Ph.D.
Oklahoma Transplantation Institute
Baptist Medical Center of Oklahoma
Oklahoma City, OK

David L. Cooper, Ph.D., M.D.
Associate Professor of Pathology
Department of Pathology
University of Pittsburgh
Pittsburgh, PA

Steven Deeks, M.D.
Assistant Clinical Professor
  of Medicine
San Francisco General Hospital
San Francisco, CA

Rebecca Dresser, J.D.
The Law School
Case Western Reserve University
Cleveland, OH

Jay A. Fishman, M.D.
Chief, Clinical Transplant
  Infectious Disease Unit
Massachusetts General Hospital
Boston, MA

Suzanne Ildstad, M.D.
Professor of Surgery
University of Pittsburgh
Pittsburgh, PA

Olga Jonasson, M.D.
Director, Education and Surgical
  Services
American College of Surgeons
Chicago, Ill

Barry Kahan, M.D., Ph.D.
Director of Immunology and Organ
  Transplants
University of Texas
Houston, TX

Michale Keeling, D.V.M.
Professor of Veterinary Medicine
  and Surgery
University of Texas Cancer Center
Bastrop, TX

Len Koch
The Health, Safety and Research
  Alliance of New York State
New York, NY

Beverly Koller, Ph.D.
Department of Medicine
University of North Carolina
Chapel Hill, NC

Susan E. Lederer, Ph.D.
Associate Professor
Pennsylvania State University
College of Medicine
Hershey, PA

Justin Leiber, Ph.D.
Professor of Philosophy
Department of Philosophy
University of Houston
Houston, TX

Brenda Lein
Project Inform
San Francisco, CA

Paul T. Menzel, Ph.D.
Interim Provost
Pacific Lutheran University
Tacoma, WA

Richard A. Merrill, L.L.B.
Daniel Caplin Professor of Law
University of Virginia School
  of Law
Charlottesville, VA

Frederick Murphy, D.V.M., Ph.D.
Dean, School of Veterinary Medicine
University of California
Davis, CA

Ali Naji, M.D.
Professor of Surgery
The University of Pennsylvania
Philadelphia, PA

David H. Persing, M.D., Ph.D.
Director
Molecular Microbiology Laboratory
Mayo Clinic
Rochester, MN

Jeffrey L. Platt, M.D.
Professor, Department of Surgery
Duke University Medical Center
Durham, NC

Jonathan Y. Richmond, Ph.D.
Director, Office of Health and Safety
Centers for Disease Control
  and Prevention
Atlanta, GA

Camillo Ricordi, M.D.
Professor of Surgery
Chief, Division of Cellular
  Transplantation
University of Miami School of
  Medicine
Miami, FL

John D. Robinson, Ed.D., MPH
Chief, Interdepartmental Treatment
  Programs
Department of Psychiatry
Howard University Hospital
Washington, DC

Andrew Rowan, Ph.D.
Associate Professor, Environmental
  Studies
Center for Animals and Public Policy
Tufts University School of Veterinary
  Medicine
North Grafton, MA

David W. Scharp, M.D.
Chief Scientific Officer
Neocrin Company
Irvine, CA

Steven Squinto, Ph.D.
Vice-President of Research and
  Molecular Sciences
Alexion Pharmaceuticals, Inc.
New Haven, CT

Thomas Starzl, M.D.
Professor of Surgery
Director
Pittsburgh Transplantation
  Institute
University of Pittsburgh
Pittsburgh, PA

M. Michael Swindle, D.V.M.
Director, Division of Laboratory
  Animal Resources
Professor and Chairman
Department of Comparative Medicine
Medical University of South Carolina
Charleston, SC

James Walters, Ph.D.
Professor of Christian Ethics
Loma Linda University
Claremont, CA

Mr. Calvin Wilkins
Rumsey Island, MD

Mrs. Evelyn Wilkins
Rumsey Island, MD

Stuart Youngner, M.D.
Department of Medicine
University Hospitals
Cleveland, OH

B

List of Participants

WORKSHOP ON XENOGRAFT TRANSPLANTATION:
SCIENCE, ETHICS, AND PUBLIC POLICY

George Abouna, M.D.
Hahnemann University Hospital
Philadelphia, PA

Bernadette Alford, Ph.D.
Alexion Pharmaceuticals
New Haven, CT

Richard C. Allen
Theracell
Flemington, NJ

Thomas Arrowsmith-Low
Human Tissue Program
Center for Biologics Evaluation
 and Research
Food and Drug Administration
Rockville, MD

Fritz Bach, M.D.
Harvard Medical School
Deaconess Hospital
Boston, MA

Stephen Badylak, D.V.M., Ph.D., M.D.
Purdue University
Hillenbrand Biomedical
 Engineering Center
West Lafayette, IN

Clyde Barker, M.D.
Hospital of the University of
 Pennsylvania
Philadelphia, PA

Rachel Bartlett
Nuffield Council on Bioethics
London, UK

Robert Bauchwitz, M.D.
Columbia University
New York, NY

Paul R. Beninger, M.D.
Division of General and Restorative
 Devices
Food and Drug Administration
Rockville, MD

Gary Bennett, Ph.D.
National Institute on Dental Research
Bethesda, MD

Alan H. Berger
Animal Protection Institute
Sacramento, CA

David Berkowitz, Ph.D.
Center for Drug Evaluation
 and Research
Food and Drug Administration
Rockville, MD

John Bishop
Consumer Safety Office
Food and Drug Administration
Rockville, MD

Robin Biswas, M.D.
Laboratory of Hepatitis
Division of Transfusion Transmitted
  Diseases
Office of Blood Research and Review
Food and Drug Administration
Rockville, MD

Lauren Black, Ph.D.
Center for Drug Evaluation
  and Research
Food and Drug Administration
Rockville, MD

Eda Bloom, Ph.D.
Center for Biologics Evaluation
  and Research
Food and Drug Administration
Rockville, MD

Nancy Blustein
Division of Allergy, Immunology,
  and Transplantation
National Institute of Allergy and
  Infectious Diseases
Bethesda, MD

Ezio Bonvini
Immunobiology Laboratory
Division of Monoclonal Antibodies
Center for Biologics Evaluation
  and Research
Food and Drug Administration
Bethesda, MD

Judith Braslow, M.D.
Division of Organ Transplantation
U.S. Department of Health and Human
  Services
Rockville, MD

Mary M. Brennan
Foundation for Biomedical Research
Washington, DC

Andrew Breslin
Animalearn
Jenkintown, PA

Sandra Bridges, Ph.D.
National Institute for Allergy and
  Infectious Diseases
Bethesda, MD

Bobby Brown, D.V.M.
National Center for Infectious Diseases
Centers for Disease Control and
  Prevention
Atlanta, GA

Ruth Bulger, Ph.D.
Henry M. Jackson Foundation
Rockville, MD

Parris Burd, Ph.D.
Center for Biologics Evaluation
  and Research
Food and Drug Administration
Rockville, MD

Lewis Burrows, M.D.
The Mount Sinai School of Medicine
New York, NY

Richard C. Daly, M.D.
Division of Thoracic and
  Cardiovascular Surgery
Mayo Clinic
Rochester, MN

Joseph Cassells, M.D
Office for Protection from
  Research Risk
National Institutes of Health
Bethesda, MD

Joy Cavagnaro, Ph.D.
Center for Biologics Evaluation
  and Research
Food and Drug Administration
Rockville, MD

Marc W. Cavaille-Coll, M.D., Ph.D.
Center for Drug Evaluation and
  Research
Food and Drug Administration
Rockville, MD

Mrunal Chapekar, Ph.D.
Center for Biologics Evaluation
  and Research
Food and Drug Administration
Rockville, MD

Dolph Chianchiano
National Kidney Foundation
New York, NY

Sang Cho, M.D.
Boston University Medical Center
Boston, MA

Charles Clifford D.V.M., Ph.D
Charles River Laboratories
Wilmington, MA

Paul Colombani, M.D., FACS, FAAP
Johns Hopkins University
Baltimore, MD

Jim Compart
Compart Management Services, Inc.
Nicollet, MN

D.V. Cramer
Cedars-Sinai Research Institute
Cedars-Sinai Medical Center
Beverly Hills, CA

Nancy Cummings
Research and Assessment
National Institute for Diabetes,
  Digestive, and Kidney Diseases
Bethesda, MD

Peter Danib, Ph.D.
Columbia University
New York, NY

Martin Delaney
Project Inform
San Francisco, CA

Henry Desmarais
Health Policy Alternatives
Washington, DC

Paul Didisheim, M.D.
Biomaterials Program
National Heart, Lung, and Blood
  Institute
Bethesda, MD

Dale Distant
Department of Surgery
State University of New York
Brooklyn, NY

Alejandro Donoso, Ph.D.
Hoechst-Roussel Pharmaceuticals
Somerville, NJ

Lee Ducat
National Disease Research Interchange
Chicago, IL

Dennis Dwyer
National SPF Swine Accrediting
  Agency
Conrad, IA

Albert Edge, Ph.D.
Director, Molecular and Cellular
  Biology
Diacrin, Inc.
Charlestown, MA

Thomas Eggerman, M.D., Ph.D.
Laboratory of Molecular and Tumor
  Biology
Center for Biologics Evaluation
  and Research
Food and Drug Administration
Bethesda, MD

Richard Ehrenreich
Columbia University
New York, NY

Gerald L. Eichinger, D.V.M., J.D.
Agency for International Development
Washington, DC

Mary Ellison, Ph.D.
United Network for Organ Sharing
Richmond, VA

Daniel M. Ferree
United Network for Organ Sharing
Richmond, VA

Donald Fink, Ph.D.
Center for Biologics Evaluation
   and Research
Food and Drug Administration
Rockville, MD

Eric A. Fischer, Ph.D.
Board on Biology
Commission on Life Sciences
National Research Council
Washington, DC

Robert A. Fisher, M.D.
Liver Transplant Program
Richmond, VA

Terrance Fisher
Charles River Laboratories
Wilmington, MA

Thomas Folks, Ph.D.
National Center for Infectious Diseases
Centers for Disease Control and
   Prevention
Atlanta, GA

Tracy Fortson
National Association for Biomedical
   Research
Washington, DC

Brad Fowler
RioCore Incorporated
Topeka, KS

Ira Fox, M.D.
Department of Surgery
University of Nebraska Medical Center
Omaha, NB

Joel Frader, M.D.
University of Pittsburgh
Children's Hospital of Pittsburgh
Pittsburgh, PA

Kenneth Franco, M.D.
Yale University School of Medicine
Department of Surgery
New Haven, CT

Nelson Garnett, D.V.M.
Office of Protection from
   Research Risks
National Institutes of Health
Rockville, MD

Bette Goldman
Center for Biologics Evaluation
   and Research
Food and Drug Administration
Rockville, MD

Robert A. Goldstein, M.D., Ph.D.
National Institute of Allergy and
   Infectious Diseases
Bethesda, MD

Janet Gonder, Ph.D.
Baxter Healthcare Corporation
Round Lake, IL

Joe Graham
Red Basket Ranch
Park City, UT

Angus Grant, M.D.
Center for Biologics Evaluation
  and Research
Food and Drug Administration
Rockville, MD

Martin Green, Ph.D.
Center for Biologics Evaluation
  and Research
Food and Drug Administration
Rockville, MD

Julia Greenstein, Ph.D.
Biotransplant, Inc.
Charlestown, MA

Ronald Gress, M.D.
National Cancer Institute
Bethesda, MD

Mark Hanson, Ph.D.
The Hastings Center
Briarcliff Manor, NY

Mark Hardy, M.D.
Columbia University College of
  Physicians and Surgeons
New York, NY

David Harlan, M.D.
Naval Medical Research Institute
Bethesda, MD

Robert Harland, M.D.
Duke University Medical Center
Durham, NC

Joan Harmon, M.D.
National Institute for Diabetes,
  Digestive, and Kidney Diseases
Bethesda, MD

John Harper, Ph.D.
Life Cell Corporation
The Woodlands, TX

Florence Haseltine, M.D., Ph.D.
National Institute of Child Health
  and Human Development
Bethesda, MD

Kenneth L. Hastings
Center for Drug Evaluation
  and Research
Food and Drug Administration
Rockville, MD

Kiki Hellman, Ph.D
Food and Drug Administration
Rockville, MD

Rose-Marie Holman
College of Physicians and
  Surgeons
Columbia University
New York, NY

Mathias Hukkelhoven
Sandoz Pharmaceuticals
East Hanover, NJ

Alvin Illig
Red Basket Ranch
Park City, UT

Silviu Itescu
Division of Cardiothoracic Surgery
Columbia University
New York, NY

Jeffrey Jacob
Research Corporation Technologies
Tucson, AZ

Harold Jaffe, M.D.
National Center for Infectious Diseases
Centers for Disease Control and
  Prevention
Atlanta, GA

Judith Jansen
College of Physicians and Surgeons
Columbia University
New York, NY

Eric Johnson, M.D.
University of Minnesota
Minneapolis, MN

Frances Johnson, M.D.
Stanford University School
  of Medicine
Stanford, CA

Jane Johnson
Planned Parenthood Federation
  of America
New York, NY

Commander Carl June, USN
Naval Medical Research and
  Development Command
Bethesda, MD

Christina Kaufman, Ph.D.
Cellular Therapeutics
University of Pittsburgh
Pittsburgh, PA

Stephen Kelley
Department of Surgery
Geisinger Medical Center
Danville, PA

Arifa Khan
Center for Biologics Evaluation
  and Research
Food and Drug Administration
Bethesda, MD

Maryanne Kichuk, M.D.
College of Physicians and Surgeons
Columbia University
New York, NY

Sara King
Juvenile Diabetes Foundation
New York, NY

Shaun Kirkpatrick
Research Corporation Technologies
Tucson, AZ

Richard Klein
Food and Drug Administration
Rockville, MD

Marianne Koch
Health, Safety, and Research Alliance
  of New York State
New York, NY

Donald Kornfeld
Columbia University
New York, NY

Lisa Kory
Transplant Recipients International
  Organization
Washington, DC

Lee Kou
Stanford University in Washington
Washington, DC

Thomas Kozma, Ph.D.
MED Institute, Inc.
West Lafayette, IN

Thomas Kresina, Ph.D.
National Institute for Diabetes,
  Digestive, and Kidney Diseases
Bethesda, MD

Leslie J. Krueger, Ph.D.
Medical College of Pennsylvania
  and Hahnemann University
Philadelphia, PA

Michael Langan
National Organization for Rare
 Disorders
Washington, DC

Elliot Lebowitz, Ph.D.
Biotransplant, Inc.
Charlestown, MA

Lisa Hara Levin, D.V.M.
Americans for Medical Progress
New Haven, CT

S. Robert Levine, M.D.
Juvenile Diabetes Foundation
New York, NY

Andrew Lewis, M.D.
Center for Biologics Evaluation
 and Research
Food and Drug Administration
Bethesda, MD

David Lilienfeld, M.D.
The EMMES Corporation
Potomac, MD

Melody Lin, Ph.D.
Human Subjects Research
Rockville, MD

John Logan, Ph.D.
Nextran, Inc.
Princeton, NJ

Jeannine Majd
Biology and Biomedical Sciences
 Division
Office of Naval Research
Arlington, VA

Dr. Leonard Makowka
Ceders Sinai Medical Center
Los Angeles, CA

Diane Maloney
Center for Biologics Evaluation
 and Research
Food and Drug Administration
Rockville, MD

Lorraine Marchand
National Institute for Diabetes,
 Digestive, and Kidney Diseases
Bethesda, MD

Ignazio Marino, M.D.
Pittsburgh Transplantation Institute
University of Pittsburgh Medical
 Center
Pittsburgh, PA

George E. Mark III
Cellular and Molecular Biology
Merck Research Laboratories
Rahway, NJ

Louis Marzella, M.D.
Center for Biologics Evaluation
 and Research
Food and Drug Administration
Rockville, MD

Judith Massicot-Fisher, Ph.D.
Division of Heart and Vascular
 Diseases
National Heart, Lung, and Blood
 Institute
Bethesda, MD

Barbara Matthews, M.D.
Center for Biologics Evaluation
 and Research
Food and Drug Administration
Rockville, MD

Peter Matthews, D.V.M.
Veterinary Consultant
Gilbert, IA

Gwen Mayes
Division of Organ Transplantation
Food and Drug Administration
Rockville, MD

Christopher McGregor, M.D.
Mayo Clinic
Rochester, MN

Priti Mehnotra, Ph.D.
Center for Biologics Evaluation
  and Research
Food and Drug Administration
Rockville, MD

Francoise Meyer, Ph.D.
Sandoz Pharmaceutical Corporation
Palo Alto, CA

Robert Michler, M.D.
Cardiac Transplantation Service
Columbia University College of
  Physicians and Surgeons
New York, NY

Joshua Miller, M.D.
Division of Transplantation
University of Miami
Miami, FL

Claude Mullon, Ph.D.
Grace Biomedical
W.R. Grace and Company
Lexington, MA

Basil Mundy II
National Kidney Foundation
New York, NY

Stephen Munn, M.D.
Mayo Clinic
Rochester, MN

Detlef Niese
Sandoz Pharmaceutical Company
Basel, Switzerland

Philip Noguchi, Ph.D.
Division of Cellular and Gene
  Therapy
Food and Drug Administration
Rockville, MD

Bjorn Norrlind, M.Sc.
Department of Transplantation
  Surgery
Huddinge Hospital
Huddinge, Sweden

Henry Oh, M.D.
St. John Hospital and Medical
  Center
Detroit, MI

Daniel O'Hair, M.D.
Columbia Presbyterian Medical
  Center
New York, NY

David Onions, D.V.M.
Department of Veterinary Pathology
University of Glasgow
Glasgow, UK

Amy Patterson, M.D.
Center for Biologics Evaluation
  and Research
Food and Drug Administration
Bethesda, MD

Anne Pilaro, Ph.D.
Center for Bilologics and
  Evaluation Research
Food and Drug Administration
Rockville, MD

Daniel Pipeleers, M.D., Ph.D.
Department of Metabolism and
  Endocrinology
Universiteit Brussel
Brussels, Belgium

Jane Pitt, M.D.
Department of Pediatrics
Columbia University
New York, NY

Raymond Pollak, M.D.
University of Illinois Hospital
Chicago, IL

Harvey Pollard, Ph.D.
Laboratory of Cell Biology
 and Genetics
National Institutes of Health
Bethesda, MD

Sulli Popilskis
Columbia University
New York, NY

Susan M. Prattis, V.M.D, Ph.D.
Northwestern University
Oak Park, IL

Raj Puri, M.D., Ph.D.
Center for Biologics Evaluation
 and Research
Food and Drug Administration
Bethesda, MD

William Ramey, M.D.
St. Luke's-Roosevelt Hospital
 Center
New York, NY

M. Shane Ray
Encelle, Inc.
Greenville, NC

Abdur Razzaque, Ph.D.
Center for Biologics Evaluation
 and Research
Food and Drug Administration
Rockville, MD

Lisa Rehm
Columbia University
New York, NY

Alise Reicin, M.D.
Columbia Presbyterian Medical
 Center
New York, NY

Richard Rettig, Ph.D.
RAND Corporation
Washington, DC

Nick Reuter, M.P.H.
Office of Health Affairs
Food and Drug Administration
Rockville, MD

Rosamond Rhodes, Ph.D.
Mt. Sinai School of Medicine
New York, NY

Charles Rinaldo, Ph.D.
University of Pittsburgh
Pittsburgh, PA

Thomas C. Ripley, Ph.D.
W.R. Grace Co.
Lexington, MA

David Robinson, M.D.
Vascular Research Program
National Heart, Lung, and
 Blood Institute
Bethesda, MD

Michael Rohr, M.D., Ph.D.
Bowman Gray School of Medicine
Winston-Salem, NC

Eric A. Rose, M.D.
Columbia Presbyterian Medical
 Center
New York, NY

Stephen Rose, Ph.D.
Genetics and Transplantation Branch
National Institute for Allergy and
  Infectious Diseases
Bethesda, MD

Joe Safron, D.V.M.
Veterinary Resources
Baxter Healthcare Corporation
Round Lake, IL

Christopher Samler
Imutran, Ltd.
Cambridge, UK

Nava Sarver, M.D.
Targeted Intervention Branch
National Institute for Allergy
  and Infectious Diseases
Bethesda, MD

Kenneth Schaffner, M.D., Ph.D.
The George Washington University
Washington, DC

Dr. William Schwieterman
General Medicine Branch
Food and Drug Administration
Rockville, MD

Dr. Kenneth Seamon
Center for Biologics Evaluation
  and Research
Food and Drug Administration
Bethesda, MD

Joan Sechler
Center for Biologics Evaluation
  and Research
Food and Drug Administration
Bethesda, MD

Marian Secundy, Ph.D.
College of Medicine
Howard University
Washington, DC

Helena Selawry, M.D., Ph.D.
Veterans Administration Medical
  Center
Memphis, TN

Mercedes Serabian, Ph.D.
Center for Biologics Evaluation
  and Research
Food and Drug Administration
Rockville, MD

Aamir Sham, M.D.
Columbia Presbyterian Medical
  Center
New York, NY

Timothy Shaver, M.D.,
Organ Transplant Service
Walter Reed Army Medical Center
Washington, DC

Judith Shizuru
Division of Hematology
Stanford University School
  of Medicine
Stanford, CA

Jay Siegel
Division of Clinical Trial Design
  and Analysis
Food and Drug Administration
Rockville, MD

S. George Simon
Corporate Development
Vivorx, Inc.
Santa Monica, CA

Lisa Skeens, Ph.D.
Baxter Healthcare Corporation
McGal Park, IL

Zaid D.J. Smith, Ph.D.
Emergency Care Research Institute
Plymouth Meeting, PA

Philip Snoy, D.V.M.
Division of Veterinary Services
Food and Drug Administration
Bethesda, MD

Glen Spaulding
Tufts University School of
  Veterinary Medicine
North Grafton, MA

Joseph Spinelli, D.V.M.
Animal Care Facility
University of California
San Francisco, CA

Nancy Stanisic
Food and Drug Administration
Rockville, MD

Raymond I. Stark, M.D.
Columbia University College of
  Physicians and Surgeons
New York, NY

Jeffrey L. Steers, M.D.
Mayo Clinic and Foundation
Rochester, MN

Kathryn Stein, Ph.D.
Division of Monoclonal Antibodies
Food and Drug Administration
Rockville, MD

Irene Stith-Coleman, Ph.D.
Congressional Research Service
Washington, DC

Peter Stock, M.D., Ph.D.
Department of Transplantation
  and General Surgery
University of California
San Francisco, CA

Steven Straus, M.D.
Laboratory of Clinical Investigation
National Institute of Allergy
  and Infectious Diseases
Bethesda, MD

Gary Striker, M.D.
National Institute for Diabetes,
  Digestive, and Kidney Diseases
Bethesda, MD

William Stubing
The Greenwall Foundation
New York, NY

Colleen Sundstrom
College of Medicine
Howard University
Washington, DC

Heidi Sykes-Gomez
Sandoz Research Institute
East Hanover, NJ

Dr. Jerry Szczerban
World Health Organization
Geneva, Switzerland

Vivian Tellis, M.D.
Transplant Program
Montefiore Medical Center
Bronx, NY

Richard Thistlethwaite, Jr., M.D., PhD
Transplant Section
Department of Surgery
University of Chicago Medical Center
Chicago, IL

Annika Tibell, M.D.
Huddinge Hospital
Huddinge, Sweden

Giovanna Tosato
Center for Biologics Evaluation
  and Research
Food and Drug Administration
Rockville, MD

Wen-Ghih Tsang, Ph.D.
Vivorx, Inc.
Santa Monica, CA

Anton-Lewis Usala, M.D.
East Carolina University School
  of Medicine
Greenville, NC

Melanie Vacchio, Ph.D.
Center for Biologics Evaluation
  and Research
Food and Drug Administration
Rockville, MD

Jacky Vonderscher
Sandoz Pharmaceutical Company
Basel, Switzerland

Karen Weiss, M.D.
Food and Drug Administration
Rockville, MD

John West, M.D.
Geisinger Medical Center
Danville, PA

David Wiersma
Research Corporation Technologies
Tucson, AZ

Carol Wigglesworth
Senior Policy Analyst
Office for Protection from
  Research Risk
National Institutes of Health
Rockville, MD

Barbara Wilcox, Ph.D.
Center for Biologics Evaluation
  and Research
Food and Drug Administration
Rockville, MD

Nancy Wilkerson
Hoechst Roussell Pharmaceuticals
Somerville, NJ

Carolyn Wilson, Ph.D.
Center for Biologics Evaluation
  and Research
Food and Drug Administration
Rockville, MD

Kathryn Zoon, Ph.D.
Center for Biologics Evaluation
  and Research
Food and Drug Administration
Rockville, MD

Lee L. Zwanziger, Ph.D.
Advisors and Consultants Staff
Food and Drug Administration
Rockville, MD

C

Immunosuppression in Allotransplantation

This appendix is based on the workshop presentation of Barry Kahan and is included here to provide the reader with background information about the key features considered in developing new immunosupressive drugs or therapies. Many new immunosuppressive medications have been developed in the past two decades for the treatment of graft rejection in allotransplantation. These medications attenuate or abolish the immune reactions responsible for rejection. The new generation of immunosuppressive drugs has significantly prolonged graft survival of kidneys, livers, hearts, and heart–lungs, among others.

The ideal immunosuppressive drug has four features: it is capable of selectivity, synergy, and specificity, and it can overcome sensitization of the recipient to the transplant. These features are described below, and examples of medication in use or under development are given. Although no single immunosuppressive is ideal, and all result in serious side effects, allograft recipients often are treated successfully with combinations of different immunosuppressive drugs.

Selectivity is achieved when the immunosuppressive's effects are restricted to the immune system, as opposed to other systems of the body. For two decades, corticosteroids and azathioprine were the mainstays of treatment for allograft rejection, but they are nonselective. Corticosteroids are anti-inflammatory agents with ubiquitous effects on musculoskeletal, endocrine, gastrointestinal, and other systems. Azathioprine is slightly more selective, but it too has deleterious hematological and gastrointestinal effects. As a nucleoside synthesis inhibitor, azathioprine acts to block cell proliferation. Lymphocytes are more vulnerable than other dividing cells, but azathioprine's effects do extend beyond the immune system. Corticosteroids and azathioprine have played important roles in nonselective immunosuppression, but they are now rarely used alone because of significant short-term and long-term effects.

The ideal immunosuppressive drug should affect not all, but only a distinct subset, of factors in the immune system. Without a high degree of selectivity, an immunosuppressive can destroy much of the recipient's immune system, rendering the patient vulnerable to infection. About 80 percent of transplant recipients suffer from at least one infection, and 40 percent of transplant deaths are attributable to infectious complications of immunosuppression. The risks of immunosuppression can be alleviated by agents that achieve a high degree of selectivity.

A new class of highly selective immunosuppressives has revolutionized allotransplantation since the early 1980s. This class of drugs, called anticytokines, interferes with the T-cell response by disrupting cytokine production. The first available anticytokine was cyclosporine, which has twice the effectiveness of azathioprine in extending kidney allograft survival. Cyclosporine inhibits T-cells from producing cytokines, such as interleukin-2, which are the intercellular signals that lead to stimulation of other immune cells to attack the graft. Cyclosporine binds to a protein in the cytoplasm of T-cells to form a complex that eventually blocks a DNA-binding protein necessary for transcription of cytokine-encoding genes.

A drug similar to cyclosporine, yet even more potent, is tacrolimus (formerly known as FK506). Tacrolimus disrupts T-cell function by also binding to a cytoplasmic protein and eventually blocking production of cytokines (although the cytoplasmic protein is not the one to which cyclosporine binds). There are major side effects: nephrotoxicity occurs in approximately 30–40 percent of patients; neurological damage can occur; and over the long term, neoplasms also occur in many patients. Tacrolimus has been effective in preventing rejection of liver, kidney, heart, bone marrow, small bowel, pancreas, lung, and skin transplants. It is generally used in conjunction with corticosteroids.

Another drug in this class is serolimus (also called rapamycin). Although still in clinical trials, it has proven effective in studies of allografting in animals by prolonging survival of rat heart, kidney, and small bowel transplants, among others. It acts not by inhibiting cytokine synthesis, but rather by interfering with intracellular signal transduction. Cytokine is still produced, but T-cells cannot respond to the cytokine signal by clonal expansion. The reason is that serolimus inhibits the G_1 buildup needed for the mitotic phase of the cell cycle (Kahan and Ghobrial, 1994).

Not only is serolimus a very selective immunosuppressive, it is also an example of a drug that works synergistically with other drugs. Synergy is the second of the four ideal features of an immunosuppressive. It refers to the combined action of two drugs whose joint effect is greater than the sum of each. In experiments on rodents and dogs the combination of serolimus and cyclosporine is so synergistic that the individual doses can be reduced at least threefold. Similar results have been achieved in human clinical trials. Reducing the dose of cyclosporine is extremely desirable because it decreases the risk of toxic side effects, including renal dysfunction, hypertension, tremor, and hirsutism. Cyclosporine and other immunosuppressives also carry the long-term risk of lymphoma.

Specificity, the third key feature of an immunosuppressive, means that the therapeutic agent is directed at a particular foreign antigen. An immunosuppressive with high specificity is one that diminishes the immune response to the graft antigen but does not diminish the immune response to other antigens such as those on viruses, bacteria, and other foreign invaders. To develop a selective immunosuppressive, the graft epitope must be identified, which represents a major challenge in drug discovery. For example, xenotransplant research has identified the terminal galactose on surface glycoproteins as the determinant of hyperacute rejection and MHC (major histocompatibility complex) Class I and II (and others) as determinants of acute rejection of both allo- and xenografts (described in Chapter 2). Identification of the epitopes of these antigens has led to the development of specific immunosuppressives that modify or abolish the donor antigen. The term "selective immunosuppression" is somewhat of a misnomer in this context because these strategies do not alter the host immune system; rather, they involve alteration of the graft to prevent an immune response by the host. Strategies that alter the graft are described in more detail in Chapter 2.

Overcoming sensitization of the recipient to the transplant is the final feature of an ideal immunosuppressive agent. Immune sensitization either occurs naturally, through preformed antibodies, or is acquired. In acquired sensitization, a second exposure to an antigen results in a more rapid and robust immune response. Either natural or acquired sensitization can lead to graft rejection and generally requires treatment with increased doses of immunosuppressives. However, increasing the dose also increases the risks of side effects. None of the available immunosuppressives effectively treats sensitization. In fact, one of the immunosuppressives in use today, OKT3, is itself subject to sensitization by the host immune system. OKT3 is a mouse monoclonal antibody directed at the CD3 antigen on host T-cells. This drug is designed to deter T-cell activation by blocking T-cell binding to antigen-presenting cells. T-cells have numerous surface markers, such as CD3, that contribute to the formation of a receptor that must bind to antigen-presenting cells before recognition and activation can occur. All antibody medications derived from animal cell lines have the potential to elicit host sensitization because of foreign epitopes. Recent advances in molecular biology have enabled scientists to "humanize" animal antibodies that could result in no, or at least decreased, sensitization of the host's immune system to antibody medication.

In summary, the ideal immunosuppressive medication selectively abolishes host immune response to the graft, without altering host ability to react to other antigens; it is synergistic with combinations of medications allowing reduction in dosage and thereby reducing side effects; it is specific for graft antigens but not for undesirable antigens from infectious agents; and it overcomes the problem of host sensitization. These goals underlie research on the identification of new, less toxic immunosuppressives.